# PHYSICAL FITNESS:

# A WAY OF LIFE

# PHYSICAL FITNESS:

# A WAY OF LIFE

**Second Edition**

## Bud Getchell

Human Performance Laboratory
School of Physical Education and Athletics
Ball State University
Muncie, Indiana 47306

**JOHN WILEY & SONS, INC.**
**NEW YORK   CHICHESTER   BRISBANE   TORONTO**

**Library of Congress Cataloging in Publication Data**

Getchell, Bud, 1934–
  Physical fitness.

  Includes bibliographies and index.
  1. Exercise. 2. Physical fitness. I. Title.
RA781.G47 1979 613.7'1 78-13094
ISBN 0-471-04037-1

Printed in the United States of America

10 9 8 7 6 5

# PREFACE

Interest in physical fitness is flourishing. Courses such as Aerobics, Basic Conditioning, and Foundations of Physical Fitness are now emphasizing the *why* and the *how* of exercise. Concern for individual differences and for developing a personalized exercise prescription is now widely advocated. Cardiorespiratory endurance is becoming the central emphasis in credible programs. Despite this increased interest and progress in developing exercise programs, none of us can take good health and physical fitness for granted, especially with today's sedentary and automated life-styles. The way to insure a lifetime of physical well-being is regular participation in exercise and sports.

This book was written to help you understand the basics of physical fitness and to provide sound information for developing a systematic program of exercise and physical activity that best fits your individual needs. It is my firm belief that an understanding of how our body responds and adapts to single and repeated bouts of exercise is essential for understanding the limits of our bodies as well as for improving the functional capacity of our heart, lungs, and muscles for the betterment of our health and well-being.

Let it clearly be understood from the beginning: It takes effort to get and stay in shape. However, exercise does not have to take the form of physical punishment. We should work out hard enough to stimulate our total body, but we should always remain within our own capabilities. My intention in this book is to show you how this can be done. The information provided should help you make rational decisions about exercise; it may even serve as the foundation for a lifetime of beneficial physical activity.

The second edition continues to emphasize and recommend activities that vigorously stimulate the heart and lungs. New material has been added to provide an up-to-date documentary on the basics of physical fitness. New to this edition are the introductory statement and a listing of major concepts for each chapter. Key words and terms are now listed and defined at the end of each chapter, and a complete glossary has been added at the end of the book. The suggested readings, intended to give you greater insight into the topics discussed, have also been updated. The book is meant to be enjoyable; it is easy to read, with illustrations designed to help you delight in the many facets of exercise and sports. An attempt has been made to use as little scientific terminology as possible to facilitate understanding the basic principles. Therefore, most scholarly documentation has been omitted. As in the previous edition, the presentation is aimed at both men and women, young and old, and particularly at the person who has been a nonparticipant in sports but who needs activity to stay healthy and fit.

The key principles of health and factors involved in establishing workable fitness standards are described at the beginning of the book. The initial emphasis is on understanding and evaluating your own exercise needs. The basics for planning a personal exercise program are explained in Chapter 4. In the subsequent four chapters, different types of physical activities are discussed in detail. The final part of the book deals with long-term concerns. The relationships between nutrition, weight control, heart disease, and exercise are explored. The final chapter describes various popular sports according to their suitability as lifetime fitness activities and offers guidelines for the beginner. Although this volume is not an encyclopedia of fitness, it is a guidebook for developing a personalized fitness program.

The material in this book is the result of my work over the years in teaching courses in fitness and training people of all ages and walks of life in the area of exercise. Years of inquiry and experimentation support the exercise theories and practical suggestions offered. I am indebted to former professors, especially Dr. Thomas K. Cureton, Jr., who provided the initial spark for me in the fascinating area of physical fitness. Thanks must go to my friends of expertise in sports medicine research, who have provided the factual knowledge for the foundation of the book. I am also grateful to the many students and older adults who have taken part in our Ball State University Physical Fitness Programs over the years. Their participation has provided me with insight into the practical applications of exercise principles. I am grateful to Jim Davis (who now has a syndicated comic strip: *Garfield The Cat*) for his artistic contributions. We have appreciated the many compliments and suggestions for refinement from users of the first edition. Grateful appreciation is also extended to all the typists, especially Jo Hains, who assisted in the revisions for the new edition.

**Bud Getchell**
Muncie, Indiana

# FOREWORD

In this book Bud Getchell calls upon his years of research and experience to emphasize the crucial role of exercise in our daily lives. It is clearer than ever that regular and vigorous physical activity is the best way to insure a long and productive life. Exercise is actually our cheapest and most enjoyable form of preventive medicine.

The statistics may be familiar, but should be repeated. Since the beginning of this century, our death rate from heart disease has tripled, although mortality figures indicate a significant reduction in deaths from heart disease over the past ten years. More than half of all the deaths that occur each year in the United States from all causes, including accidents, violence, and disease, result from cardiovascular ailments. Furthermore, heart disease is a phenomenon not only of old or middle age; it begins early in life. In a recent study of eight- to twelve-year-old boys, more than half of them had at least one of the factors known to increase the risk of a heart attack in adults. In addition, autopsies of American combat fatalities in both Korea and Vietnam showed that over 70 percent of the soldiers had substantial narrowing of one or more coronary arteries, a condition traditionally associated with old age. This was true even though their average age was only 22 years! Obesity, too, has become a national problem. It is estimated that one out of five teenagers and one of three adults are grossly overweight.

Clearly, one major culprit is our increasingly sedentary life-style. It is really paradoxical. Technology has eliminated much of the heavy drudgery from our daily lives. Jobs that once demanded hours of hard labor are now automated. These advances in technology were intended to improve the quality of life. But growing evidence suggests that we are unable to adapt to a sedentary existence. Physical inactivity may actually be a major cause both of coronary artery disease and obesity. The solution, as Dr. Getchell makes abundantly clear, is a lifetime of vigorous physical activity.

In this book exercise is considered a reward not a punishment. Through his experience in establishing exercise programs for people of all ages, Dr. Getchell knows the factors that mean success or failure in developing beneficial exercise habits. After examining the concept of physical fitness and its physiological basis, he offers detailed tests and guidelines to enable the reader to evaluate his or her own physical fitness. These standards provide a sound basis for planning a personal exercise program and for measuring its continuing success. Programs for developing strength, cardiovascular endurance, flexibility, and general muscle tone are all described in detail. They are followed by a look at more advanced conditioning methods. Also, many myths about the exercise response in women are dispelled. Part III of the book deals with the interrelationships between nutrition, weight control, coronary artery disease, and physical activity. In the final chapter a wide variety of popular sports is described, with emphasis on their value and feasibility as lifelong physical fitness activities.

This second edition includes an introductory statement for each chapter, providing a brief summary of the major concepts to be presented in the chapter. A listing and definition of key words or concepts are provided at the end of each chapter, as well as in a glossary at the end of the book. Each chapter has been revised to include a discussion of recent advances in the field subsequent to the first edition. These changes and additions make this text the best of its kind for anyone interested in physical fitness. Dr. Getchell's enthusiasm is catching. Armed as well with his knowledge and advice, the reader is well on the way to a more healthy and satisfying way of life. As a finisher in the 1978 Boston Marathon, Dr. Getchell is himself an example of the joys and benefits of being physically fit.

**Jack H. Wilmore**
Professor of Physical Education
University of Arizona
Tucson, Arizona

# CONTENTS

**PART I    A BASIS FOR PHYSICAL FITNESS**

**ONE.    PHYSICAL FITNESS FOR EVERYONE                          4**

Why Physical Fitness?                                                7
What is Physical Fitness?                                            8
Fundamental Reasons for Physical Fitness                           14

**TWO.    UNDERSTANDING PHYSICAL FITNESS                        20**

Basic Structure of the Body                                        21
The Cardiorespiratory System                                       21
Exercise and Your Heart                                            24
The Training Effect on the Heart                                   25
Aerobic Capacity                                                   31
Field Tests for Aerobic Fitness                                    32
Anaerobic Capacity                                                 34
How Vigorous Exercise Benefits You                                 33
Physiological Sex Differences                                      39
Gynecological Considerations                                       40
Concluding Remarks                                                 41

**THREE.    APPRAISING YOUR FITNESS                             46**

Physical Fitness Test Battery                                      49
Interpreting Your Results                                          49
Evaluating Muscular Strength and Endurance                         51
Flexibility Evaluation                                             57
Motor Skill Evaluation                                             60
Evaluating Your Cardiorespiratory Endurance                        65
Analysis of Body Fat and Body Build                                77
A Final Word on Measurement and Evaluation                         86

FOUR.     A PRESCRIPTION FOR FITNESS                          92

          Prescription Factors                                93
          Varying Intensity, Duration, and Frequency          100
          It takes Effort to be Physically Fit                100
          Designing a Personal Program                        101
          Related Considerations                              104
          There is No Need to Hurry                           109


PART II   DEVELOPING A PROGRAM FOR PHYSICAL
          FITNESS

FIVE.     INDIVIDUALIZING CONDITIONING EXERCISES              116

          Developing a Pleasing Body Contour or Physique      117
          Basic Conditioning Exercises                        120
          A Suggested Warm-up Routine                         148
          Additional Exercises for Women                      149
          Low Back Pain                                       155
          Concluding Remarks                                  158

SIX.      CONDITIONING FOR CARDIORESPIRATORY
          ENDURANCE                                           162

          A Basic Program: Jog-Walk-Jog                       163
          Bicycling                                           170
          Swimming                                            174
          Walking                                             177
          Stationary Bicycle Exercisers                       178
          Rope Skipping                                       181
          Canoeing, Rowing, Cross-Country Skiing              183
          Concluding Remarks                                  185

SEVEN.    WEIGHT TRAINING                                     188

          Improving Strength                                  190
          A Weight Training Program                           192
          Isokinetics                                         202

EIGHT.    ADVANCED CONDITIONING METHODS                       206

          Interval Training                                   207
          Continuous Training                                 210

Continuous Versus Interval Training 211
Circuit Training 213

**PART III ADDITIONAL CONCERNS RELATED TO PHYSICAL FITNESS**

NINE. NUTRITION, WEIGHT CONTROL, AND EXERCISE 220

Nutrition Basics 222
National Dietary Goals 227
Basics for a Nutritious Diet 228
Overweight and Obesity 237
The Role of Exercise in Weight Control 240
A Plan for Losing Weight 249
Lifetime Concept of Weight Control 251

TEN. ACTIVITY AND HEART DISEASE 256

Atherosclerosis 258
Coronary Risk Factors 259
What is Your Risk? 267
Cardiac Rehabilitation 269
Physical Activity: A Preventive Measure 269

ELEVEN. A LIFETIME OF SPORTS PARTICIPATION 276

A Look at Sports and Physical Fitness 277
Lifetime Sports 278
Rating the Fitness Potential of Lifetime Sports 310
Presidential Sports Award Program 312
Fitness and Sports: Lifetime Concerns 313

**Epilogue** 320

**APPENDIX** 323

**T-Scores: Women** 324-326
**T-Scores: Men** 327-329
**Body Composition Chart** 330
**Physical Fitness Profile Charts** 331-332

**GLOSSARY** 333
**INDEX** 345

# PART ONE

# A BASIS FOR PHYSICAL FITNESS

# chapter one

It seems appropriate before studying physical fitness that a rationale for fitness be established. In order to appreciate the role of regular exercise as an integral part of your daily life-style, it is imperative to discuss why regular exercise is needed in a modern technological society. In addition, because of the many ill-supported definitions and misconceptions about physical fitness, we need to define just what is physical fitness. In short, this chapter attempts to lay the groundwork for understanding the philosophy of this book. We hope you will be encouraged to read on and consider adopting some of our suggestions for developing and maintaining a level of physical fitness that is well within your potential.

As you read this chapter give thought to the following statements:

• Exercise is something that is good for you. To be physically fit does take effort (yes, some sweat), but keep in mind that exercise does not have to be punishing to lead to and maintain optimal fitness.

• Regular and vigorous stimulation (exercise) of the total body is a necessary ingredient to muscular and circulatory health, and well-being.

• Our modern life-style fosters unfitness as technological advances tend to eliminate physical exertion from everyday activities.

• Everyday activities, even for the laborer, no longer adequately stimulate the heart, lungs, and muscles to produce physiological benefits.

• Physical fitness is a capability of the heart, blood vessels, lungs, and muscles to function at optimal efficiency.

• The basic health components of physical fitness are cardiorespiratory endurance, strength, muscular endurance, and flexibility.

# physical fitness for everyone

The better you understand the potential benefits of exercise and realize your physical capabilities and limitations, the better able you are to embark on a pattern of living that includes daily participation in stimulating and beneficial exercise.

Through no fault of your own, your present attitude toward exercise may be negative. Past physical education or athletic experiences may have created this outlook. We call it *physical miseducation.* Do you recall being punished with exercise? Have you ever been chosen last on a pick-up team? Or have you ever been ridiculed because of poor skills? For many youngsters in their growing years, physical education experiences of this type have had a negative effect. The use of calisthenics or running laps to punish a group is absolutely ridiculous. Heckling the relatively inept performer in a physical education class is inexcusable. Exercise is something

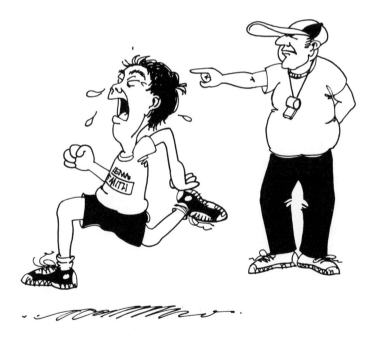

*Do you recall being punished with exercise?*

that is good for you; it is not to be used for punishment or embarrassment. It is no wonder that so many people do not participate in sports or exercise. They associate these experiences with hurt, pain, fatigue, and embarrassment.

In addition, throughout the early school years, exercise and sports programs for girls have been limited, if not excluded from the curriculum. Boys have always been encouraged to exercise, but physical exertion for girls was considered "unladylike." It is time for women not to apologize for participating vigorously in physical activities. There is no known medical reason why women should be limited in physical activities. Women respond to vigorous physical training in the same way that men do. In fact, research shows that the responses of the two sexes to vigorous activity are more similar than different.

The American Alliance for Health, Physical Education and Recreation emphasizes the necessity for individualized instruction, aimed at assisting students to find themselves physically. Traditionally, athletics have tended to develop varsity competitors for the entertainment of a physically inept society. By contrast, this book is written to help you discover your own physical resources. It is written for everyone, especially for people who may not win a championship or make the team. Why should you be merely a spectator?

You deserve an opportunity to develop skills and the fitness adequate for a full and abundant life. If you know your capabilities and limitations and understand the values of exercise, the better your chance of becoming a regular participant in physical fitness and sports activities.

Attitudes are learned through personal experiences. Many attitudes have been formed early in life and once formed may be difficult to change. Most likely, you have been brought up in an environment that is constantly seeking an easier life-style with minimal physical exertion. The need for regular exercise as a necessary ingredient to health and well-being is the theme of this book. However, simply reading this book is not enough. You need to actually get involved physically if you are to realize and understand the purpose of physical fitness. You must be willing to get involved with some of the programs suggested in this book if you are truly to reap benefits from them. At the same time, participating in a physical fitness program will give you insight into the physiological operation of your body; it will reinforce what you learn from your reading. The aim of this book is to provide guidelines for a positive and successful physical fitness experience. Ultimately, the success of this book will depend on your willingness to study the guidelines and theoretical aspects of fitness and to participate vigorously in the recommended activities.

## WHY PHYSICAL FITNESS?

Although the most opportune time for developing lifelong fitness habits is in the childhood years, it is in the late teens and early twenties when a fitness consciousness among men and women is realized. At this stage in life you have reached physical maturity; your body is at its natural peak of physiological efficiency and health. However, observe friends in their late twenties and early thirties. In many of them this natural fitness has begun to disappear. Lack of exercise is beginning to show its effect. An increase of body fatness, a loss of muscle tone, and a lessened breathing capacity are some of the obvious signs of physiological deterioration. According to Dr. Thomas K. Cureton, a renowned physical fitness expert, these middle-aged characteristics begin to reveal themselves in many Americans in their mid to late twenties.

Our modern life-style fosters unfitness. Many technological advances are intended to eliminate physical exertion from everyday activities. The automobile and television are key contributors to our sedentary life-style, and we have become accustomed to other automated energy savers: elevators, riding lawnmowers, motorized golf carts, power steering, and power windows on automobiles. At the same time, our competitive society is characterized by pressing domestic problems, business obligations, and deadline tensions. These types of stresses are interconnected with the physiological systems of the body and appear to affect one's state of health. The point is that your emotions, nerves, glands, and mental state along with your heart, lungs, and muscles are all fused into a complex, wonderful organism—your body.

Many men and women feel that their daily work provides them with enough exercise for fitness. Running up and down stairs or standing all day at a job seems to be physical exertion. It is exertion, of course, but such limited activities do not use the lungs fully, nor provide adequate stimulation for the heart to produce a training effect. If normal, day-to-day activities leave you fatigued at the end of the day, then you need the increased energy and vitality that comes from regular physical exertion. You need to use energy to gain energy. In other words, regular stimulation of the total body through vigorous exercise produces increased strength and endurance, and characteristics associated with good health. These attributes cannot be acquired from sitting at a desk all day, watching sports on televi-

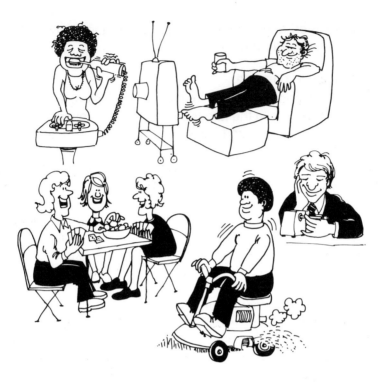

*Our modern life-style fosters unfitness.*

sion, riding elevators, or snacking on a hamburger, french fries, and a thick shake.

With inactivity recognized as a menace to physiological well-being, some authorities suggest that exercise may be the cheapest preventive medicine in the world. Researchers in medicine, nutrition, psychology, physiology, and physical education agree that physical fitness exertion is necessary for maintaining a functional physical fitness. No responsible physical educator will ever suggest that exercise is a panacea. But it is clear that, just as we need food, rest, and sleep, we need daily vigorous exertion for the maintenance of our physical capacities. Physical fitness is not an end in itself but a means to an end. It provides us with a basis for optimal physiological health and the capacity to enjoy a full life.

## WHAT IS PHYSICAL FITNESS?
Most authors define physical fitness as the capacity to carry out everyday activities (work and play) without excessive fatigue and with enough energy

in reserve for emergencies. Emphatically, this definition is inadequate for our modern way of life. By such a definition, almost anyone can classify himself as physically fit. The banker, the merchant, the nurse, or the student can probably run a city block to catch a bus, run up a flight of stairs to be on time for class, or even swim a hundred yards to shore from a capsized boat. Nevertheless, it seems risky to accept such a definition when we consider recent medical literature concerning the effects of inactivity on our health and well-being.

For example, inactivity has been identified as one of the risk factors of coronary heart disease and related cardiovascular diseases. These diseases of the heart and blood vessels are associated with a decreased blood supply to the vital areas of the body. According to the American Heart Association, the United States has the highest death rate from cardiovascular disease of any nation in the world. Autopsy studies comparing people of highly affluent nations with undeveloped countries have led many medical authorities to suspect that the differences in diet, smoking, levels of physical activity, and other living habits common to our Western society contribute to diseases of the heart and blood vessels. (See Chapter 10, "Activity and Heart Disease" for a more detailed coverage of this topic.)

In addition, the modern man or woman does not live at an optimal fitness level. Most of us are satisfied just to make minimal exertions. Repeatedly physiological studies throughout the United States bear these conclusions out. Longitudinal studies have shown a decline of physical fitness with age. However, they also positively show that this plight can be favorably slowed and changed by rational fitness training three or four days per week. This lack of optimal fitness is the result of our inactive life-style that tends to make us sluggish, lazy, and just plain unfit. In addition, we eat rich food that is high in cholesterol, fat, sugar, and calories. In many cases this diet contains too many calories, which turn into unsightly ripples of fat. However, a reasonable physical fitness program based on individual needs and interests is a very logical solution for overcoming the harmful health effects from living in a highly mechanized and technical society. You probably do not need a high level of physical fitness to work in a world dominated by technical innovations but regular physical activity is a necessity if your body is to function properly.

**Physical Fitness Defined**
Physical fitness is the capability of the heart, blood vessels, lungs, and muscles to function at optimal efficiency. Optimal efficiency means the

most favorable health needed for the enthusiastic and pleasurable participation in daily tasks and recreation activities. Optimal physical fitness makes possible a life-style that the unfit cannot enjoy. To develop and maintain physical fitness requires vigorous effort by the total body. However, the results are well worth the exertion and sweat required.

You might ask: Why do I need cardiorespiratory endurance? Or why do I need an increase in strength? The answers are the same whether you are a man or woman. It is foolish to live at your minimal potential. You need to have more than the minimal capacity for exertion to do your job and to meet emergencies. Functional cardiorespiratory and muscular systems enable you to carry out everyday activities efficiently. In other words, people who are physically fit look better, feel better, and possess the good health necessary for a happy and full life. The possession of optimal strength, muscle tone, and endurance, not only for emergencies, but for everyday living can be the key to dynamic health.

## Basic Components of Physical Fitness

Strength, muscular endurance, flexibility, and cardiorespiratory endurance are the basic components of physical fitness. These four characteristics are all equated with the healthy functioning of the body. Another trait, motor skill performance, is often cited as a fifth fitness component. It roughly means general athletic skill. We recognize the interrelationship of skill to the other aspects of fitness; however, our main concern will be with basic health components. A rating of "good" in all of these areas indicates an acceptable level of physical fitness. Chapter 3, "Appraising Your Fitness," will assist you in determining your present fitness status. For now, each component will be briefly defined to clarify its role in physical fitness.

### *Strength*

Strength is probably the most familiar component of fitness. It is the capacity of a muscle to exert a maximal force against a resistance. Strength training results in some enlargement of the muscle fibers (hypertrophy) and a relative increase in one's ability to apply force.

Strength is fundamental to all sports. A lack of reasonable strength obviously contributes to poor performance in sports. Strength often seems to be lacking in the upper arms and shoulder region, especially in women. This lack of strength directly impairs one's ability to swing a golf club or strike a tennis ball.

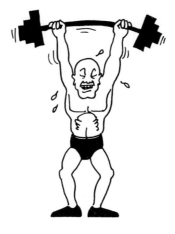

*Strength*

Properly conducted weight resistance programs (such as working with barbells) are the most efficient means for gaining rapid strength. In men such training may also result in increased bulk; to date, however, there seems to be no similar gain in bulk in women. In Chapter 7 we explain the reasons for this lack of muscle enlargement in women and discuss weight training techniques for the development of strength.

### Muscular Endurance
This trait is often used synonymously and incorrectly with strength. Endurance is the capacity of a muscle to exert a force repeatedly over a period of time. Also, it refers to the ability of the muscle to hold a fixed or static contraction for a period of time. In other words, it is the ability to apply

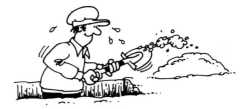

*Muscular endurance*

strength and sustain it. Your ability to do sit-ups or pull-ups is an indication of your <u>muscular endurance.</u> The capacity of your legs to carry you beyond a distance of two miles, of your arm to repeatedly pitch a baseball, or of your hands consistently to grip a golf club firmly are also examples of muscular endurance. Even activities around the home, such as shoveling snow, washing windows, painting, and cleaning house, all require some degree of prolonged muscular exertion.

### *Flexibility*

<u>Flexibility</u> is the ability to use a muscle throughout its maximum range of motion. It is your ability to move your joints—to bend, stretch, and twist them easily.

Stand up and place your feet together. Now bend down slowly and touch your fingertips to the floor. Do you feel a tightening of the muscles at the back of your thighs? If so, these muscles need stretching. They need greater flexibility. It is advantageous to possess a full range of motion at the various major joints of the body. Maintenance of good joint mobility provides increased resistance to muscle injury and soreness. Short muscles may become sore muscles when subject to physical exertion. Inflexible joints and muscles limit movement. For example, the need for flexibility varies with your specific needs. In swimming, shoulder and ankle flexibility are important for efficient movement through the water. In karate the muscles of the legs, arms, and abdomen need a full range of movement. In fact, graceful movements in walking and jogging require some degree of elasticity of the major muscle groups.

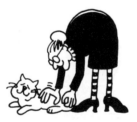

*Flexibility*

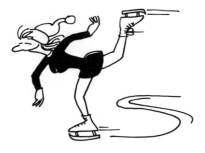

*Motor skill performance*

### Motor Skill Performance

Although a desirable attribute, having a high degree of motor skill (athletic ability) is not essential for maintaining a good level of physical health. Your own ability to dodge, to control your balance, to react and move quickly, and the ability of your muscles to function harmoniously and efficiently are all reflections of your general athletic skill. The ability of the nerves to receive and provide impulses that result in smooth coordinated muscular movements is a wonder of the human body. It is evident in the flawless performance of the great athletes.

Motor skill can usually be evaluated with simple tests. The vertical jump (requiring explosive power), an agility run (requiring speed, balance, and agility) and squat thrusts (requiring speed of body movement) have traditionally been used as tests of motor skill and general athletic ability. Such tests have always been popular for the athletically inclined.

### Cardiorespiratory Endurance

Although the physical fitness characteristics given above are important, they are more effectively linked to the strength of the heart and lungs. Cardiorespiratory endurance *is the most essential physical fitness component.* Your life depends on the capacity of your heart, blood vessels, and lungs to deliver nutrients and oxygen to your tissues and to remove wastes. Efficient functioning of the heart and lungs is required for optimal enjoyment of such activities as jogging, swimming, cycling, and many of the vigorous sports presented in this book.

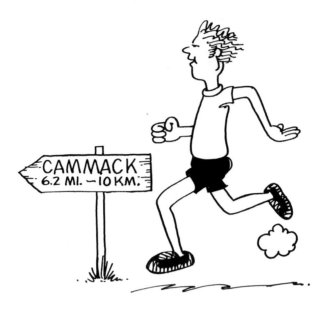

*Cardiorespiratory endurance*

## FUNDAMENTAL REASONS FOR PHYSICAL FITNESS

Over the years two fundamental reasons have been established for undertaking a physical fitness program. First, vigorous exercise results in muscular and cardiorespiratory health. Second, and more generally, physical fitness enhances the capacity to enjoy life fully. Throughout this book, a sincere attempt will be made to explain how a good fitness program suits these purposes.

### Optimal Muscular and Cardiorespiratory Health

It is a physiological fact that the human organism needs stimulating exercise. When your total body is subjected to regular muscular activity, requiring a vigorous stress on the heart, lungs, and muscles, the general efficiency of your physiological functions improve. There is no scientific evidence showing harmful effects from regular exercise in a healthy person. But an abundance of research now strongly supports the theory that regular, vigorous exercise helps keep healthy hearts healthy and may prevent cardiovascular disease.

For example, the fit person adjusts to increased physical demands and

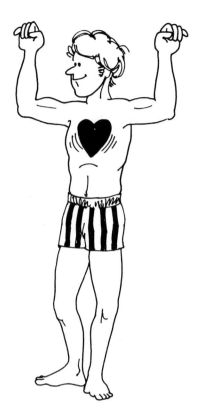

*Optimal muscular and cardiorespiratory health*

returns to a normal state more quickly than the unfit person. A physically fit heart beats at a lower rate and pumps more blood per beat at rest. As the result of regular exercise an individual's capacity to use oxygen (this means the ability to do more physical work) is increased substantially. Although regular exercise is not a cure-all, it is a sound means for maintaining a high level of health.

**Enjoying a Full Life**
People who keep fit greatly enlarge their fullness of living. They can do a day's work with ease; they can meet most emergencies; and they can extend their recreational activities to a second set of tennis, an extra nine holes of golf, or a hike on a trail.

Today, more and more people are becoming interested in individual activities and sports. Recreations such as backpacking, hiking, cross-country skiing, scuba diving, bicycling, and jogging are growing in popularity. However, to give complete enjoyment, participation in these activities

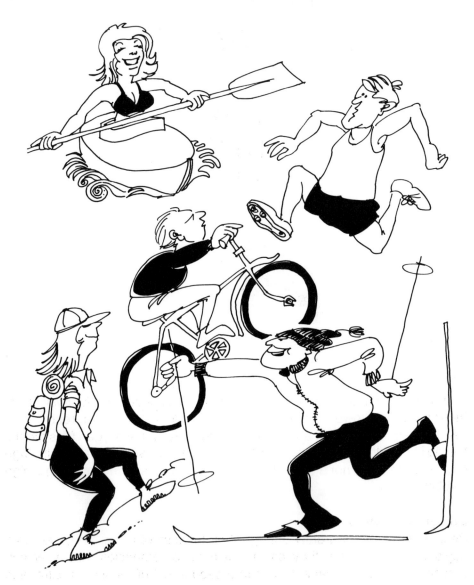

*People who keep fit greatly enlarge their fullness of living.*

require a level of physical fitness beyond that needed in everyday life. To be pleasurable a hike up a mountain or a scuba dive in a lake require adequate physical conditioning. In other words, to enjoy your recreational endeavors fully, you need to be in shape.

Being physically fit provides the robust health and the available excess energy needed to fully appreciate the joys of life. Simply put, it means doing more with quality. We don't necessarily exercise to arrive at an increased physical capacity to enjoy a full life. Being able to do more things with competency and pleasure makes for healthy and enjoyable living.

## KEY WORDS

CARDIORESPIRATORY ENDURANCE: The capacity of your heart, blood vessels, and lungs to function efficiently during vigorous, sustained activity such as jogging, swimming, and cycling.

FLEXIBILITY: The range of movement of a specific joint and its corresponding muscle groups.

MOTOR SKILL: The ability of muscles to function harmoniously and efficiently, resulting in smooth coordinated muscular movement. A reflection of general athletic skill.

MUSCULAR ENDURANCE: The capacity of a muscle to exert a force repeatedly or to hold a fixed or static contraction over a period of time.

STRENGTH: The capacity of a muscle to exert a force against a resistance.

## SUPPLEMENTARY READINGS

Alley, Louis, "Focus on the Quality of Life," *Journal of Health, Physical Education, and Recreation.* 42:8–10, September, 1971.

Astrand, Per-Olof, "Do We Need Physical Conditioning." *Journal of Physical Education.* Special Edition: 129–136, March–April, 1972.

Cooper, Kenneth, *Aerobics.* New York: Evans, 1969.

Cureton, Thomas K., *Physical Fitness and Dynamic Health.* New York: Dial, 1965.

Fixx, James F., *The Complete Book of Running*. New York: Random House, 1977.

Graham, M.F., *Prescription for Life*. New York: McKay, 1966.

Harris, Dorothy V., "Dimensions of Physical Activity." *Women and Sport: A National Research Conference*. Dorothy V. Harris, ed., Pennsylvania State University, 1972, pages 3–15.

Higdon, Hal, *Fitness After Forty*. Mountain View, California: World Publications, 1977.

Holland, George J. and Elwood C. Davis, *Values of Physical Activity*. Third edition, Dubuque, Iowa: Brown, 1975.

Kennedy, John F., "The Soft American." *Sports Illustrated*. December 26, 1960.

McCloy, Charles H., "What is Physical Fitness?" *Journal of Health, Physical Education and Recreation*. **27**:16–17, September, 1956.

Nash, Jay B., "Contributions and Relationships of Health, Physical Education and Recreation to Fitness." *Anthology of Contemporary Readings*. Second Edition, Dubuque, Iowa: Brown, 1970, pages 29–40.

# chapter two

In this chapter we will discuss the fundamental workings of the heart, lungs, and muscles and how these organs respond to exercise. A basic understanding of these phenomena will help you to understand the complexities of physical fitness as well as to acquire an appreciation of how the body responds favorably to vigorous exercise.

You will learn how the heart, blood vessels, and lungs function jointly as the cardiorespiratory system to provide blood loaded with oxygen and nutrients to the cells of the body for energy. In addition, this chapter summarizes the potential benefits of regular exercise including benefits specific to women.

As you read this chapter give thought to the following statements:

• It is well-accepted that the overall physiological functioning of the body will benefit if the body is properly stimulated on a regular basis with exercise. In contrast, disuse of the body readily results in a decline of the vital functions for good health and well-being.

• The heart is a phenomenal muscular pump that is vital to life. Exercise, properly done, strengthens the heart and improves its ability to function *better* during everyday living.

• Oxygen is needed for life. The ability of the body to use oxygen depends on the capacity of the cardiorespiratory system to function efficiently. The proper exercise will improve and maintain the body's ability to use oxygen.

• Laboratory methods can be used for measuring the functional capacity of your cardiorespiratory system, often referred to as maximal oxygen uptake or aerobic capacity. Running tests sustained for over 10 minutes such as a 2-mile or 1.5-mile run have correlated quite well with the more sophisticated lab measures for measuring maximal oxygen uptake, a key measure of physical fitness.

• Maximal oxygen uptake measurement is universally accepted as a prime indicator of one's functional level of cardiorespiratory fitness.

# understanding physical fitness

It is universally accepted that the physiological functions of the body improve with use and decline with disuse. More specifically, the heart, lungs, and muscles become stronger and more durable the more they are used. To understand the complexities of physical fitness, we need a fundamental knowledge of human physiology and of the mechanisms involved in developing and maintaining physical fitness. This chapter provides a very simple explanation of the physiology of exercise, the effects of exercise on the body, and other essentials for a better understanding of physical fitness.

## BASIC STRUCTURE OF THE BODY

The smallest structural and functional unit of the body is the *cell.* Cells are found in countless sizes and shapes. High-powered microscopes are required to study the smallest cells, whereas the human egg cell can be seen by the unaided eye. Protoplasm, the jellylike material that is the basic substance of all cells, is the medium in which complex biochemical tasks are continually carried out.

Groups of cells joined together to perform a similar function are termed *tissues.* Combinations of different kinds of tissue form *organs.* And organs unite to form a unit of organization called an *organ system.* For example, various kinds of tissue such as nerves, muscles, and connective tissue, are found in the heart. The heart, an organ, is part of the circulatory system. Muscles, another system, attach to bones and span joints and activate these mechanical levers to make movement possible. The nervous and endocrine (glandular) systems control the functioning of the body. Nerves conduct impulses throughout the body. They control muscle movement and other vital functions. Hormones or chemical messengers also help control the body's activities.

## THE CARDIORESPIRATORY SYSTEM

The maintenance of life depends on efficient operation of the body at the cellular level. Each cell needs a ready supply of oxygen, and food, while carbon dioxide and other waste products must be carried away from it. Adequate functioning of the circulatory and respiratory systems is needed for these life-sustaining services. The cardiovascular system (the heart and blood vessels) keeps the blood circulating throughout the body. The respiratory system (the lungs and air passages) removes carbon dioxide and replaces it with fresh oxygen. Because of their dependence on each other, the two systems are often referred to jointly as the cardiorespiratory system. Healthy functioning of the cardiorespiratory system is of paramount importance.

## The Blood
The blood is the fluid that flows through the circulatory system. This aqueous medium is a slurry of blood cells, foodstuffs, minerals, gases, and many other substances that are vital to the proper functioning of the body. For example, the blood transports nutrients (foods) and oxygen to the tissues. From the tissues it carries away cellular waste products and distributes the heat generated from the activities of the cell. Approximately 45 percent of the blood volume is composed primarily of red blood cells, white blood cells, and platelets. The remainder is a liquid called plasma. The red blood cells are composed of iron-protein molecules called hemoglobin. Hemoglobin combines readily with oxygen and carbon dioxide and, when the situation demands, will easily give up these molecules. The plasma is a complex liquid consisting of food, minerals, hormones, and chemical substances needed by the cells for coordinating and regulating cellular functions.

An artery is an elastic vessel that carries blood away from the heart. A vein returns blood to the heart from the tissues. In the systematic circulation, (that is, all blood vessels aside from the heart and lungs) the arteries carry oxygen and nutrients to the tissue cells of the body. These cells receive their fuel and oxygen through thin-walled structures called capillaries that are distributed throughout tissues of the body. Carbon dioxide and other end products are picked up in these tissues and carried back in the veins to the right atrium of the heart.

## The Heart
The heart beats constantly. It pumps blood throughout the body at approximately 72 beats per minute, or 100,000 beats per day. It circulates at least 2000 gallons of blood a day. This powerful muscular pump never fails, and we usually assume it won't. After you climb up a flight of stairs, your skeletal muscles relax, but your heart keeps on beating.

The heart is composed of two upper chambers called atria and two lower chambers called ventricles (Figure 2.1). The right atrium and the right ventricle are separated from their counterparts on the left by a muscular wall. This separation allows the heart to work as two separate pumps (right and left). In addition, each atrium is connected to its corresponding ventricle by a oneway valve. The right side receives blood from the body that is low in oxygen and pumps it to the lungs. At the same time, the left side receives fresh, oxygenated blood from the lungs and pumps it out through the aorta, the largest artery in the body, to all tissues of the body.

Contrary to what you might expect, the blood passing through the chambers of the heart does not nourish the heart muscle. Instead, arterial branches called coronary arteries which originate from the aorta, direct blood over the outer surface of the heart through numerous branches. These branches divide into smaller arteries and capillaries in the cardiac (heart) muscle. In this way each cardiac muscle fiber receives nourishment. The blood is then returned to the right atrium through the coronary sinus, a large vein formed by the coronary veins.

The heart rate, and the amount of blood pumped from the heart with each beat, varies with the changing needs of the body. At rest the heart

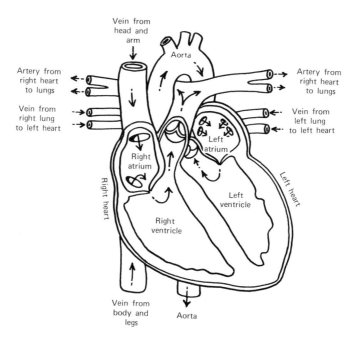

*Figure 2.1   The heart*

pumps about five liters (1 liter equals 1.06 quarts) of blood a minute. But it is capable of increasing this output to 15 to 25 liters of blood a minute when the body is active.

## The Lungs

The lungs, located within the rib cage, are the organs of respiration that regulate the exchange of the air between the blood and external environment. Air enters the body by either the nose or mouth. It then passes into the throat, which is also a passageway for food. The throat branches into two tubes, the esophagus through which food passes to the stomach and the trachea through which air passes to the lungs. The trachea extends downward toward the lungs. It divides into two branches called bronchi, one leading to each lung. Within each lung each bronchus divides and subdivides throughout the entire organ. Eventually, this subdivision ends in tiny ducts attached to an estimated one billion microscopic air sacs called alveoli. These air sacs are clustered together, giving the lungs a spongy texture. Blood capillaries surround the alveoli.

When air is breathed into the lungs, the oxygen molecules pass through the walls of the alveoli into the capillaries. There they combine with molecules of hemoglobin, a protein-iron pigment in the red blood cells. From the lungs, this oxygenated blood returns to the heart, which pumps it to all parts of the body. Throughout the body oxygen is picked up by the cells that need it, and the blood in turn picks up carbon dioxide and other waste products. This carbon dioxide is returned by the venous system (veins) to the heart and then to the lungs where it is given up and eventually breathed out through the nose and mouth.

At rest the lungs breathe in about six to eight liters of air each minute. This rate increases during the mildest exertion. The amount of increase depends upon the intensity and the duration of the exertion. While walking, climbing stairs, jogging, or playing basketball, for instance, the cells require more oxygen. Breathing increases in both depth and rate. The level of ventilation may reach well over 100 liters a minute in an all-out athletic performance. Correspondingly, the oxygen requirement ranges from a quarter of a liter at rest to a maximum of three to five liters or more.

## EXERCISE AND YOUR HEART

Vigorous participation in activities such as basketball, swimming, or jogging increases the cells' need for oxygen. Accordingly, it also increases the levels of waste products to be removed from them. The working cells have to receive an increased blood flow. The heart must pump faster, and it must increase its stroke volume, that is, its volume for each beat.

An inability to get enough oxygen and the buildup of carbon dioxide, a waste product, hinders the ability of the muscles to contract. But it is well known that the lungs always contain ample oxygen for the circulating blood to pick up as it passes through them. Furthermore, the oxygenated blood leaving the lungs and returning to the heart is almost always saturated with oxygen. (That is, the blood is holding all the oxygen it can.) The problem, therefore, is to get more blood to the active muscle tissue to meet the requirements of exertion. This need can be met by increasing the speed with which the blood goes through the circulatory system.

For instance, an activity requires three liters of oxygen a minute, but the heart is able to pump only enough blood to supply two liters of oxygen per minute for this task. In a very short time, the buildup of metabolic wastes (carbon dioxide and lactic acid) in the cell and the shortage of oxygen will reduce the capacity for movement. Eventually movement will have to stop. In short, your muscles are fatigued. From this example, you can easily recognize the importance of the heart's ability to pump large amounts of blood during exercise.

In some people, the heart's capacity to transport blood and deliver oxygen to the tissues is limited. It is unable to pump sufficient blood in time of stress. The feeling of being "out of breath" or exhausted during exercise is not due to a shortage of oxygen in the lungs. Rather, it results from the inability of the heart to pump sufficient blood to the muscle tissues. The functional ability of your heart to pump blood and of your muscle fibers to utilize oxygen are the keys to successful muscular performance.

## THE TRAINING EFFECT ON THE HEART
The term training effect describes the many physiological changes that result from participation in vigorous muscular fitness activities. As you progress in a conditioning program, the training effect on your heart will begin to show. The heart rate varies with the activity you are performing. An increased heart rate is accompanied by an increase in the amount of blood pumped per beat (the stroke volume), and the magnitude of the stroke volume depends on the functional strength of the heart. It is a physiological fact that the regularly exercised heart will improve its performance. As the result of systematic training, the heart will be able to pump more blood per beat.

## Heart-Rate Response During Exercise

As exercise begins, the heart rate increases. The elevation in heart rate is directly proportional to the work load (Figure 2.2). In other words, as the work load is gradually increased, the heart rate also increases. (Note the closed circles in Figure 2.3.) Tests were made on a group of sedentary college men. Walking at 3.5 mph (a brisk walking speed) for three minutes elevated their hearts to an average of 129 beats per minute. Jogging at 7.5 mph (the pace of an eight-minute mile), for three minutes resulted in a mean heart rate of 185 beats per minute. When the running speed was increased to 8.6 mph (a seven-minute mile) the heart rate rose even higher, to 194.

Over the years, heart-rate responses to standardized work loads have served as convenient indicators of physical fitness capacities and changes. Figure 2.3 illustrates the mean changes in these same college men after eight weeks of training. The training consisted of a progressive jog-walk-jog program of two 20-minute periods a week. The working heart rate at each selected speed is clearly lowered. For example, regular exercise lowered the walking heart rate to 110 beats a minute. But the heart rate is still high compared with that of a top university cross-country runner facing the same work loads. This is also illustrated in Figure 2.3. The increase in heart rate from its resting level is less in the better-conditioned individual while performing the same work.

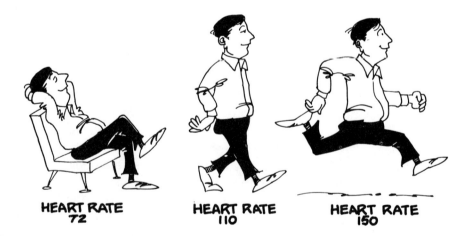

**HEART RATE**
**72**

**HEART RATE**
**110**

**HEART RATE**
**150**

*Figure 2.2   The heart rate increases in direct proportion to the work load.*

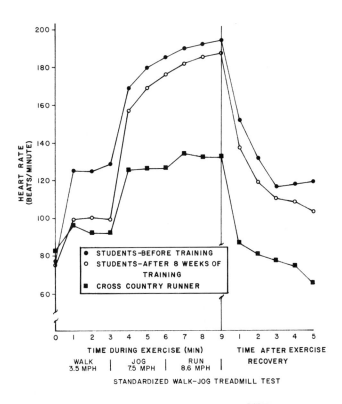

*Figure 2.3    Heart-rate response during exercise and recovery*

**Heart-Rate Response During Recovery**
A more rapid recovery of the heart rate after a workout also indicates cardiac efficiency. In Figure 2.3 note the corresponding recovery rates of the students and the cross-country runner. In summary, the physically fit person generally has a lower heart rate and a more rapid recovery time for any given exercise work load.

**Maximal Heart Rate**
The increase in heart rate is in direct proportion to the increase in work load, up to a limit. But when you perform very strenuous exercise to the point of exhaustion, you reach your maximal heart rate. This is your highest attainable heart rate. Maximal heart rates of 180 to 200 beats per minute have been observed in young people with some values of higher than 220 beats per minute reported. At any given maximal heart rate, the heart with

the largest capacity per beat (the largest stroke volume) will pump the most blood. That is, it will reach the highest cardiac output. (Cardiac output is the product of stroke volume and heart rate.) The larger the stroke volume, the higher the heart's ability to do work and the higher the level of performance.

## Aerobic Capacity

Human beings need oxygen to live. The ability of the body to utilize oxygen depends on the functional efficiency of the cardiorespiratory system: the lungs, the heart, the blood vessels, and the associated tissues. During vigorous activity, the exercising muscles use increased amounts of oxygen and produce corresponding amounts of carbon dioxide.

The largest amount of oxygen that you can consume per minute is called your maximal oxygen uptake. This maximal value, often referred to as your aerobic capacity, is a functional measure of your physical fitness. The maximum effort you can exert over a prolonged period of time is limited by your ability to deliver oxygen to the active tissues. Theoretically, a higher oxygen uptake indicates an increased ability of the heart to pump blood, of the lungs to ventilate larger volumes of air, and of the muscle cells to take up oxygen and remove carbon dioxide.

Regular vigorous exercise will produce a training effect that can increase your aerobic capacity by as much as 20 to 30 percent. The precise amount of increase depends on your pretraining status and on the intensity and duration of your training program.

In the laboratory, the body's ability to use oxygen can be measured during exercise (Figure 2.4). A common instrument for regulating the work load is the treadmill. It is a motor-driven conveyer belt, constructed so that the speed and the angle of incline are adjustable. To perform the test one walks or jogs on the belt.

During a treadmill stress test, the subject's volume of expired air is measured, and samples of this air are analyzed for their oxygen and carbon dioxide content. The analysis is made by biochemical or, more recently, electronic methods. If we know the volume of air breathed and its oxygen and carbon dioxide content, we can calculate the amount of oxygen consumed by the subject. By exercising the subject to his highest level (when he can do no more), we can determine his aerobic capacity, or maximal oxygen uptake. This value is universally accepted as an indicator of physical fitness. Not only does it measure the functional ability of the heart and lungs, but it also measures the cell's capacity to utilize the oxygen delivered to it by the blood.

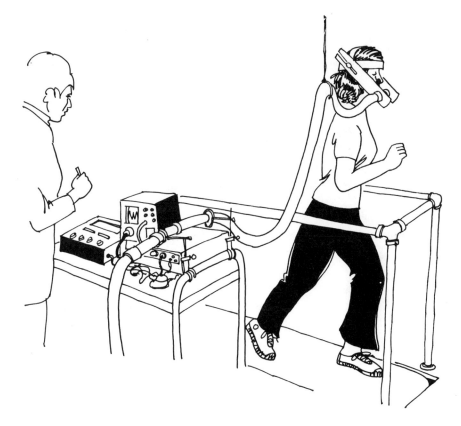

*Figure 2.4   Measuring aerobic capacity during a treadmill stress test*

Maximal oxygen uptake is usually expressed as the amount of oxygen (expressed in milliliters) that can be consumed for each kilogram of body weight. (A kilogram is 2.2 pounds.) The highest aerobic capacity ever recorded was measured in a male cross-country skier: 94 ml/kg•min. The highest female value, 74.0 ml/kg•min, also belonged to a cross-country skier. Champion marathoners have been found to have values of about 75 to 82 ml/kg•min. Recently we tested a group of runners (40 plus years) who qualified for the Boston Marathon. Their measured aerobic capacities were between 58 and 62 ml/kg•min.

The average aerobic capacity for an untrained college male, as determined by many studies, is between 42 and 46 ml/kg•min. College women, untrained, appear to fall between 30 and 39 ml/kg•min. Figure 2.5 shows

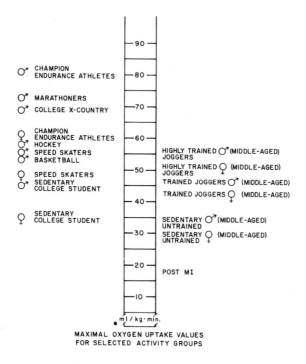

CHAMPION
ENDURANCE ATHLETES ♂

MARATHONERS ♂
COLLEGE X-COUNTRY ♂

CHAMPION
ENDURANCE ATHLETES ♀
HOCKEY ♂♀
SPEED SKATERS ♂♀
BASKETBALL ♂♀

SPEED SKATERS ♀
SEDENTARY ♂♀
COLLEGE STUDENT

SEDENTARY ♀
COLLEGE STUDENT

90
80
70
60
50
40
30
20
10

HIGHLY TRAINED ♂ (MIDDLE-AGED)
JOGGERS

HIGHLY TRAINED ♀ (MIDDLE-AGED)
JOGGERS

TRAINED JOGGERS ♂ (MIDDLE-AGED)

TRAINED JOGGERS ♀ (MIDDLE-AGED)

SEDENTARY ♂ (MIDDLE-AGED)
UNTRAINED

SEDENTARY ♀ (MIDDLE-AGED)
UNTRAINED

POST MI

ml / kg · min.

MAXIMAL OXYGEN UPTAKE VALUES
FOR SELECTED ACTIVITY GROUPS

*Figure 2.5*

the relative maximal oxygen uptake position for some male and female athletes and some middle aged joggers. The middle-aged values indicate that, to some extent, your position on the fitness continuum can be controlled by physical training. It must be pointed out, though, that the maximum position an individual can reach in aerobic capacity also depends on such factors as heredity, age, and sex.

Therefore, the maximal oxygen uptake scale reflects the capacities of a range of individuals, from athletes of superior endurance (e.g., cross-country runners and marathoners) to sedentary and inactive people. The lowest figure on the scale represents the average value for people who have recently suffered a heart attack or myocardial infarction ("Post MI" on the graph).

It is important to realize that shortly after you reach adulthood (ages 18 to 21) your aerobic capacity begins to decline gradually. The decrease is greater in inactive and overweight people, and in those who have de-

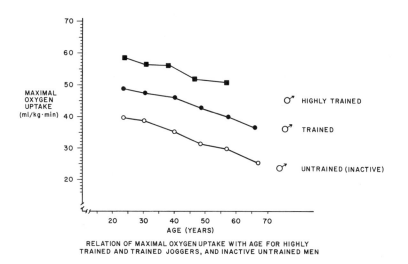

RELATION OF MAXIMAL OXYGEN UPTAKE WITH AGE FOR HIGHLY
TRAINED AND TRAINED JOGGERS, AND INACTIVE UNTRAINED MEN

*Figure 2.6*

veloped diseases of the heart and lungs. Growing evidence indicates that a regular exercise program can delay this decline.

In Figure 2.6 we see that maximal oxygen uptake gradually declines with age. The graph presents recent data from our lab for men. Regardless of one's training status, there is a natural decline with age. However, note the higher levels of physical conditioning for the trained men. The lowest slope represents sedentary, inactive men prior to engaging in a jog-walk-jog fitness program. The middle slope (moderately trained) represents men who have had at least 10 weeks of training and who jog six to 14 miles a week (a minimum of one and one-half to two miles per session). The highly trained group comprises men who train faithfully at 15 to 30 miles per week (a minimum of three miles per session). The gradual decline in maximal oxygen capacity with age seems to hold true for women also, although the data at this time are limited.

## FIELD TESTS FOR AEROBIC FITNESS

Obviously, it is not possible to measure everyone's heart rate during exercise in the laboratory, nor is it feasible to measure the oxygen functions of the heart and lungs. For this reason, field tests, (tests outside the laboratory) have been devised that measure performance. For example, the speed with which you can run distances of one and one-half or two miles or the distance you can cover in a selected time period, such as 12 minutes, are good field tests for aerobic fitness. Research has demonstrated that these running tests correlate highly with maximal oxygen uptake. The person who is in better physical condition should be able to run two miles in a faster time or cover a greater distance in 12 minutes than the more poorly conditioned person. A minimum distance of one and a half miles or a time period of 12 to 15 minutes has been established as the minimum for adequately estimating your aerobic capacity. To date, it is not known whether these tests are reliable indicators of oxygen uptake capacities for sedentary, untrained people. However, they are an easy means for indicating the relative level of aerobic capacity in a person who has progressed in a training program. Chapter 3 deals with a more comprehensive appraisal of fitness. It includes these tests for estimating your maximal oxygen uptake and assessing your aerobic fitness level.

## ANAEROBIC CAPACITY
The previous section dealt with the role of oxygen in prolonged muscular exertion. Your aerobic capacity reflects the fullest possible use of your potential for taking up oxygen. At times, however, high-speed intense work of short duration requires immediate energy that cannot be attained quickly enough from aerobic sources. In this situation, another process, termed anaerobic metabolism, is called on for a ready supply of energy. Anaerobic means "without oxygen", thus, anaerobic energy is the output of energy when the oxygen supply is insufficient.

### The Chemistry of Muscle Contraction
All cells derive their energy for life from an energy-rich substance called ATP (adenosine triphosphate). This compound is always present in the cell and provides energy for muscle contraction, for the transportation of vital substances through the cell membrane, and for the reforming and breakdown of chemical compounds in the cell. After ATP is broken down and used, there is a need to reform it. When oxygen in the cell combines with a foodstuff (for example, sugar) energy is produced to restore the ATP supply. At times, especially during short, exhaustive exercise, an ample supply of oxygen isn't available in the muscle. Thus, other mechanisms are needed to rebuild ATP immediately. One of these processes is the use of CP (creatine phosphate). The major role of the CP stores in the cell is to reload the ATP for muscular contraction. However, in a few seconds this mechanism (CP supply) is exhausted. The other means of quick energy

when oxygen is lacking is the breakdown of glycogen (stored sugar) to lactate, which can also supply energy for muscle contraction. This process extends the ability of the muscle to contract, until an accumulation of lactic acid becomes so great that the contraction stops. These events are called the anaerobic phase of muscle chemistry because no oxygen is required. For contractions to continue, oxygen is needed and the sugars are broken down in a process called the Krebs cycle. The final end products of this cycle are carbon dioxide, water, and energy, which is released for the purpose of restoring CP and ATP. During this oxidative process, 18 times more energy is released than during the anerobic phase. Usually in most types of exercise the anaerobic and aerobic processes take place simultaneously.

**Relationship of Aerobic and Anaerobic Energy**
Such high-energy activities as short sprints and sudden bursts of activity are examples of anaerobic activities. High-performance athletic feats are more apt to require an anaerobic fitness and a basic aerobic capacity. In contrast, physical fitness programs for health and wellbeing do not require

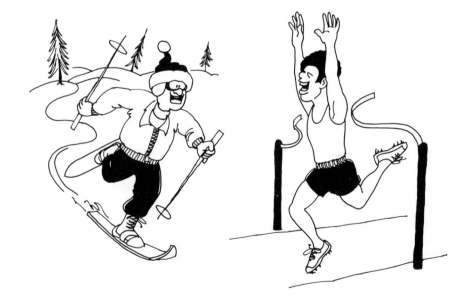

*Prolonged exercise—aerobic*                    *Short bursts of exercise—anaerobic*

substantial anaerobic development. During prolonged exercise (e.g., walking and jogging), most of the energy is aerobic, derived from the oxidation of carbohydrates and fats. However, during the early stages of exercise and during short bouts of exercise the energy is anaerobic, derived from the splitting of energy-rich substances stored within the muscle cell without oxygen.

Oxygen's function is to restore the cell's energy-rich substances such as ATP (adenosine triphosphate) and CP (creatine phosphate). When the oxygen supply cannot meet the energy requirement, the muscle fatigues; eventually it is unable to continue working. The extent to which the anaerobic processes are activated can be found in the laboratory by measuring the blood lactate concentrations.

## HOW VIGOROUS EXERCISE BENEFITS YOU

Some of the immediate, more noticeable effects of vigorous exercise are deep breathing, profuse sweating, and a rapid beating of the heart. These changes from rest occur whether you are in shape or not. However, if you continue to exercise vigorously on a regular basis (day by day and week by week) some changes will gradually take place. These changes occur as a result of adaptation of the body to exercise, and are referred to as the training effect of exercise, which we previously defined. Total body exercise will affect the entire body; however, some areas are helped more than others. Our purpose here is to briefly summarize some of the beneficial effects of exercise on the body.

### Cardiorespiratory Benefits

After a period of training (six to eight weeks) there is a slow but consistent reduction in the resting heart rate along with an increase in stroke volume. Since this means that more blood is pumped with each heart beat, the heart does not have to beat as often to supply the body with blood. In addition, the slower heart rate and increased stroke volume provide a greater rest for the heart between beats.

Strenuous training will stimulate dramatic improvements in exercise performance (e.g., in a two-mile run time) and maximal oxygen uptake (aerobic capacity). Training studies have shown that aerobic capacity is directly related to improved stroke volume and cardiac output during prolonged work. In addition, people with high aerobic capacities have the potential for a greater perfusion of blood in the exercising muscles. Recent research from muscle biopsies has shown that there is an increase in the

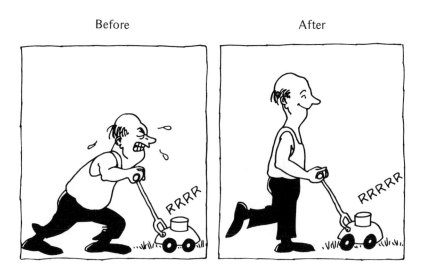

*Cardiorespiratory benefits*

amount of enzymes needed for muscular contraction following consider-able aerobic training. Finally, it is well established that aerobic capacity is related to the ability to perform prolonged exercise.

Several studies have indicated that active people tend to have lower resting blood pressures than more sedentary people. However, for people who have already acquired serious medical complications related to high blood pressure, the benefits of exercise for lowering blood pressure may be limited.

The evidence on the effects of exercise on the concentration levels of the two major fat substances in the blood is encouraging. These fats, choles-terol and triglycerides, are believed to be involved in heart disease. The research suggests that the less these substances are present in the blood serum the better. People who are very active and who adhere to sound nutritional practices tend to have lower concentrations of these fats in their blood. (Chapter 10 discusses this subject in greater detail.)

**Body Composition Benefits**
Exercise programs directed at building strength and flexibility will facilitate the formation of firm and supple muscles. An increase in muscular strength is related to an enlargement of the muscle fibers, that is, an increase in muscle mass. However, in women this increase in muscle fiber thickeness

Before                    After

*Body composition benefits*

is not as great as in men. (A more comprehensive discussion of strength development can be found in Chapter 7, "Weight Training.")

People who possess a good to high level of physical fitness are seldom overweight or, more important, they tend not to be fat. Many studies have shown that body fat is reduced as the result of vigorous, regular training. Exercise is the great variable in weight control. (Chapter 9 explains the role of exercise in controlling your body weight.)

At present it seems that in the early stages of a training program there is little weight loss. Instead, the body composition is redistributed and firmed up. In other words, muscles get stronger, and increase in mass, and fat disappears from the storage depots. Consequently, body weight remains the same even though there is a fat loss. In most cases, weight loss during the first weeks of training is the result of dieting.

## Psychological Benefits

Among the most beneficial outcomes of vigorous activity are the psychological benefits. Although the evidence is not clear-cut, a sense of calm is one result of participating in exercise, according to many active people. Sports and exercise as a diversion from the everyday duties of work provide excellent relief and relaxation for the mind and body.

Before After

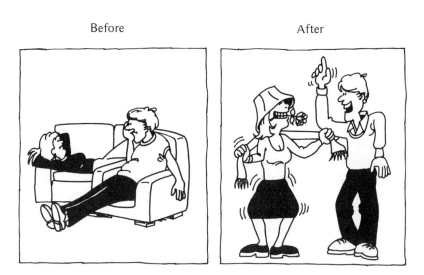

*Psychological benefits*

Dr. Ronald Lawrence, founder and president of the American Medical Joggers Assocation, is convinced that vigorous exercise, in this case jogging and running, improves your total well-being. He feels you sleep better but require less sleep. Your sex life is enhanced. You are better prepared to cope with stress and improve your work productivity. Whether these benefits are classified as physical or mental, he keenly feels that vigorous activity strengthens one's quality of life.

Dr. George Sheehan, a cardiologist and runner, who recently wrote a best seller *Running and Being,* asserts that it is the psychology of fitness that is important rather than the physiology of fitness. According to Dr. Sheehan, "Play is our most important product." One who plays is fulfilling himself and becoming the person he is. Dr. Sheehan recommends that you first become a good animal, know your body, and enjoy it. It is then that you discover play and fun. For him, running is an hour of play and enjoyment away from his daily routine.

Although George Sheehan's words refer mainly to running, it seems reasonable to assume that exercise or "play" can also provide a great "high." It can refresh the soul and provide a mental release; most important, people who exercise regularly feel more alive. Dr. Kostrubala, a San Diego Psychiatrist, has had remarkable results treating his patients by having them run. This form of therapy has had profound mental effects on them. Depression was eased, medications abandoned, smoking and drinking reduced or eliminated, and their general overall well-being improved. Dr. Kostrubala suggests that vigorous physical activity such as running may cause some body chemistry reaction that helps to restore emotional stability.

Dr. Kenneth Cooper of the Aerobics Institute feels strongly that people who are physically fit often tend to be psychologically fit. They exhibit a "fitness glow"—that is, they do feel better, they do look better, and they do have an improved self-image. Cooper suggests that once a person becomes physically fit he feels better, because he is more relaxed, more in tune, more aware, and more perceptive.

In summary, most physical fitness advocates feel that there is a definite relationship between physical, mental, and spiritual well-being. Perhaps the physiological benefits are like a bonus, and the feelings and mental "highs" that come from being physically active and fit are the true benefits.

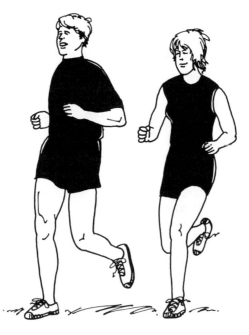

*Research suggests men and women respond similarly to exercise.*

## PHYSIOLOGICAL SEX DIFFERENCES

To date, much of the physiological data on women have been generalized from the results of investigations on men. The standards of excellence in sports and physical fitness achievement have been based on male performances and any achievement falling short of these standards has been interpreted as inferior. Whether or not the female's physiological response to exercise is limited by sex has not been determined. Research is beginning to suggest, however, that the responses of both sexes to vigorous physical activity are much more similar than different.

Sedentary middle-aged women and men were recently compared following a 10-week exercise program. Although the women had lower values for maximal oxygen uptake, their rate of improvement was similar to that of the men. Exercise heart rates also improved (that is, decreased) proportionately with those of the men. Loss of skinfold fat at selected sites was also comparable. Thus, even though sexes differ in body size and structure, when these differences are allowed for, their responses to vigorous exercise are essentially the same.

Many women fear that vigorous exercise will make them heavily muscled and unfeminine-looking. There is no scientific evidence to substantiate this fear. Women normally have less muscle mass than men. However, the development of muscle mass is as varied among women as it is among men. Thus, some women may be stronger and faster than some men. The inherent capacity for muscle development, however, is genetically determined by the sex hormone levels. The male hormone, testosterone, is responsible for muscle bulkiness in males. This hormone is present in women, but in amounts that are probably too low to have a substantial effect on muscle size. In Chapter 7 "Weight Training" a more detailed discussion on muscle bulk in women is presented.

According to Dr. Joan Ullyot, a physician and running enthusiast, women are different from men in their physical endowment. In general, women have less muscle mass than men (23 percent compared to 40 percent muscle mass of a man's body), have a lighter bone structure, and have more body fat than men. Thus, for people of the same height, a woman will usually weigh less than a man, and she will have less power to propel the same mass.

There have been recent claims that women naturally burn fat as muscle fuel and perhaps may be more suited to endurance performance. To date, no laboratory evidence exists to substantiate this theory. However, we do know that endurance training does assist the working muscles for the more efficient use of fat for energy. As for a women's physiology having an advantage over men in long races and endurance-type events, there seems to be no scientific basis for such a claim.

A woman cannot carry as much oxygen in her blood as men (that is, she has a lower aerobic capacity), a factor that may limit her endurance. This is because women generally have fewer total red blood cells and about 15 percent less hemoglobin (the protein-iron molecule that carries oxygen in their blood) when compared to men. In women this combination of a small muscle mass, fewer red blood cells, and a lower hemoglobin means that men have a greater potential for endurance. Nevertheless, both men and women must exert effort in training, but the amount of effort must be determined individually. This topic will be covered in greater detail in Chapters 4 and 6.

## GYNECOLOGICAL CONSIDERATIONS

For years there have been many contradictory assertions about the relationship of physical activity to female physiological phenomena such as the menstruation cycle, pregnancy, and childbirth. The extent to which these events are affected by physical conditioning is still not certain. Nevertheless, at the very least, it appears that regular, vigorous exercise does not have any deleterious effect on women's physiology.

### Menstruation

There are probably more myths about menstruation than about any other area of female sexuality. For years it was traditional for girls to excuse themselves from physical education class during their menstrual periods. Today, there is disagreement among medical authorities as to the wisdom of vigorous exercise during the menstrual period. Scientific evidence is limited, but surveys and interviews of women athletic performers have provided some insights. A recent article in *womenSports* summarized the latest information and clearly suggests that the normal routine of life should not be interrupted during menstruation. The athletic performance of some women may suffer during premenstrual or early menstrual days. However, women have won Olympic medals during every phase of the menstrual cycle. Moreover, simply worrying about the effect of menstruation will have a detrimental influence on performance.

Since the menstrual period is a normal physiological function, if a woman feels well during her period, she may continue her regular exercise habits. Overtraining, however, may lead to a deviation from the normal rhythmic pattern. Thus, it is wise to maintain an accurate record of menstrual cycles. If deviations occur, medical advice should be sought.

**Pregnancy and Childbirth**
The literature is also very limited in providing reasonable exercise guidelines for pregnant women. Heavy training for athletic competition, especially during the final three months of pregnancy, has been frowned upon. However, for a woman who has been physically active before conception, continuation of her exercise program during pregnancy seems permissible. The fetus is well-cushioned, floating in a sack of fluid that acts as a shock absorber. Such activities as walking, jogging, and cycling cannot harm the baby. In contrast, engaging in springboard diving, gymnastics, judo, and similar activities is risky.

Most authorities recommend that a woman continue her normal physical fitness activities, though taking care not to become overfatigued. In fact, this is sound advice for anyone in a physical fitness training program, pregnant or not. There is no need to overdo it; this will be constantly emphasized throughout this book. Beginning a program of physical conditioning at the onset of pregnancy, however, might be unwise. "Crash" exercise programs during pregnancy cannot substitute for long-term regular physical conditioning. If you choose to begin a program during pregnancy, you should seek medical consultation and supervision from an authority on exercise.

Women who have athletic backgrounds or who are habitually active tend to have a smaller incidence of complications during pregnancy as well as quick and easy deliveries. This is because of their good cardiorespiratory system, muscle control, and abdominal muscle tone. Women with strong abdominal muscles can speed labor for the simple reason that they can really bear down hard during delivery. In general, women who possess a high degree of physiological fitness appear not be bothered as much with the most common gynecological problems as the women who are unfit.

**CONCLUDING REMARKS**
It is hoped that this chapter has helped you to better understand the physiological basis for exercise and physical fitness. We have intentionally avoided complex scientific terms. Our purpose has been to provide some fundamental understanding with emphasis on the mechanisms involved during physical exercise. In conjunction with this basic knowledge, we reviewed the benefits that can result from participating in vigorous exercise on a regular basis.

The better you understand the basic facets of physical fitness, the better your chance of becoming actively involved in some of the sports and exercise programs that we discuss in this book. For people who wish a more sophisticated background in exercise physiology, readings in textbooks devoted entirely to this subject are recommended. We have described physical fitness in simple terms and have not written a comprehensive chapter on the physiology of exercise. This is because an extensive background in physiology is not needed to understand the basics of physical fitness. However, the material presented in this chapter is essential for a better understanding of the chapters to follow.

## KEY WORDS

AEROBIC CAPACITY: A functional measure of physical fitness based on the measurement of maximal oxygen uptake. Generally synonymous with terms maximal oxygen uptake and cardiorespiratory endurance.

ANAEROBIC: Means "without oxygen" and refers to the output of energy for muscular contraction when the oxygen supply is insufficient.

ARTERY: An elastic vessel that transports blood away from the heart.

BLOOD PRESSURE: The force that blood exerts against the walls of the blood vessels and that makes the blood flow through the circulatory system.

CAPILLARIES: The smallest vessels in the circulatory system where all exchanges of nutrients and respiratory gases takes place between the blood and tissues.

CARBON DIOXIDE: The waste gas given off during the breakdown of foodstuffs in the cell and transported in the blood to the lungs and exhaled.

CARDIAC OUTPUT: The amount of blood pumped by the heart per minute. The product of stroke volume times the heart rate.

CORONARY ARTERIES: Refers to the arteries that supply blood and nourishment to the heart muscle.

FIELD TESTS: Refers to physical fitness tests performed outside the controlled environment of the laboratory (e.g., 2-mile run, sit-ups).

GLYCOGEN: The form in which carbohydrates are stored in the muscles and liver.

HEART: A powerful muscular pump responsible for blood circulation.

HEART RATE: Refers to the number of times the heart beats per minute. In most cases the number of heart beats each minute is equal to the number of pulse beats per minute.

LUNGS: Located within the rib cage, these two organs regulate the exchange of air between the blood and external environment.

MAXIMAL HEART RATE: The highest attainable heart rate for an individual.

MAXIMAL OXYGEN UPTAKE: The largest amount of oxygen that can be consumed per minute. It is the best physiological index of cardiorespiratory endurance. Often referred to as maximal aerobic capacity, maximal oxygen intake, or maximal oxygen consumption.

MENSTRUATION: The periodic cycle in the uterus of the female associated with preparation of the uterus to receive a fertilized egg.

OXYGEN: The essential respiratory gas for life processes in the cell.

STROKE VOLUME: The volume of blood ejected from the left ventricle during one heart beat.

TRAINING EFFECT: The term used to describe the many physiological changes that result from participation in vigorous, muscular fitness activities.

TREADMILL: A testing device consisting of a motor-driven conveyor belt constructed so that the speed and angle of incline can be regulated to produce varying workloads.

TRIGLYCERIDES: Fat particles that are stored in the body. Also they provide the main means by which fat is transported in the blood. Recent evidence has revealed an association with atherosclerosis (see CHOLESTEROL).

VEIN: A vessel that carries blood back to the heart.

VENTRICLE: The chamber of the heart that pumps blood to the lungs (right ventricle) or to all the systems of the body (left ventricle).

## SUPPLEMENTARY READINGS

Astrand, Per-Olof and Kaare Rodahl, *Textbook of Work Physiology.* Second Edition, New York: McGraw-Hill, 1977.

Buskirk, E. R., "Cardiovascular Adaptation to Physical Effort in Healthy Men." *Exercise Testing And Exercise Training In Coronary Heart Disease,* John Naughton and Herman Hellerstein, eds. New York: Academic, 1973.

Drinkwater, Barbara, "Maximal Oxygen Uptake of Females." *Women and Sport: A National Research Conference,* Dorothy V. Harris, ed. Pennsylvania State University, 1972, pages 375–386.

Fox, E. L. and D. K. Mathews, *The Physiological Basis of Physical Education and Athletics.* Second Edition, Philadelphia: Saunders, 1976.

Glasser, William, *Positive Addiction.* New York: Harper & Row, 1976.

Harris, Dorothy, "Women in Sports: Some Common Misconceptions." *Journal of Sports Medicine.* 1:15–17, March-April, 1973.

Kostrubala, Thaddeus, *The Joy of Running.* New York: Pocket Books, 1977.

Nagle, Frank S., "Physiological Assessment of Maximal Performance," *Exercise and Sports Sciences Reviews,* Vol. 1, Jack Wilmore, ed. New York: Academic, 1973.

Saltin, Bengt, "Physiological Effects of Physical Conditioning," *Medicine and Science in Sports.* 1 (1), March, 1969.

Shaffer, Thomas E., "Physiological Considerations of the Female Participant," *Women and Sport: A National Research Conference.* Dorothy V. Harris, ed., Pennsylvania State University, 1972, pages 321–331.

Sheehan, George, *Running and Being.* New York: Simon and Schuster, 1978.

Ullyot, Joan, *Women's Running.* Mountain View, California: World Publications, 1977.

Weber, Ellen, "The Three Great Myths of Sex and Sport." *womenSports.* **2**:30–33, January, 1975.

Wilmore, Jack H., *Athletic Training and Physical Fitness: Physiological Principles and Practices of the Conditioning Process.* Boston: Allyn and Bacon, 1976.

# chapter three

How do you know whether you are fit? This chapter is intended to help you to evaluate your physical fitness. Such an evaluation will provide you with insight into your strengths and weaknesses. Also, a basis for setting personal fitness goals can be gained from these measurements, and later on the effectiveness of your individualized training program can be determined.

The tests selected measure the basic components of physical fitness and can be administered with ease and consistency. The tests represent the major areas of fitness: muscular strength and endurance, flexibility, cardiorespiratory endurance, and motor skill performance. Although physical fitness tests have limitations, these recommended tests will provide you with a rough estimate of your physical fitness status. Norm tables are provided for rating your results.

In addition, procedures are recommended for assessing your body fat and body build. From these data you can compute a desired weight.

As you read this chapter give thought to the following statements:

• Testing should not dominate your exercise program. Physical fitness measurements, however, will not only help you in evaluating your present condition, but assist you in setting reasonable goals.

• Physical fitness is individual. The intent of self-testing is to help you evaluate the effectiveness of your training program.

• For persons over 30, or anyone who has not recently been active, a medical exam is recommended before attempting these vigorous tests or any exercise program.

• In order to gain an all-inclusive evaluation, tests representing traits from each of the physical fitness components should be utilized.

• Field tests such as 2-mile or 1.5-mile run correlate very well with the laboratory-determined values for maximal oxygen uptake (aerobic capacity).

• It is the proportion of fat tissue in your body rather than your scale weight that determines your desirable weight.

# appraising your fitness

Physical fitness means more than bulging muscles or a trim waistline. A lean appearance, although desirable, does not necessarily reflect your physical fitness. No matter how you look, or even how strong you are, you have a low level of fitness if your heart is unable to meet the circulatory demands of prolonged work. Many men and women, for instance, appear very trim but tire easily while carrying out their everyday activities.

Each individual is unique, with different abilities in various physical and mental skills. In addition, all people have their own physiological limitations. Therefore, evaluating physical fitness is a very complex matter. This chapter is designed to assist you in developing a practical testing program for appraising your fitness strengths and weaknesses.

It is a fundamental aspect of human nature to be curious of how we compare with others. Physical fitness measurements afford you the opportunity to evaluate your physical status. Most important, they give you a basis for setting personal goals and they enable you to test the effectiveness of your training program.

Recently, the use of physical fitness tests has been criticized because they totally disregard specific physical factors. Test results have traditionally been interpreted without consideration of individual differences. Yet factors such as body build (weight, height, fatness) and anatomical differences can adversely affect one's performance on physical fitness tests. For example, a 150-pound man may be able to complete eight pull-ups whereas a 200-pound man can only get his chin over the bar four times. How do you compare these results when one man is pulling up an extra 50 pounds? Both physical fitness tests and the norm tables that have been developed from testing large groups of people who share these limitations.

Nevertheless, despite the shortcomings of physical fitness tests and norms, it seems worthwhile to appraise your body's abilities, whether it weighs 250 pounds or only 135 pounds. Regardless of the norms, how many times can you pull your body weight over the chinning bar? What is your estimated aerobic capacity, based on your jogging ability? Are you flexible, and how much can you improve your flexibility? These questions are the reasons for measurement. How do you rate on the fitness components and can you improve on your weaknesses?

Physical fitness testing should not dominate a conditioning program.

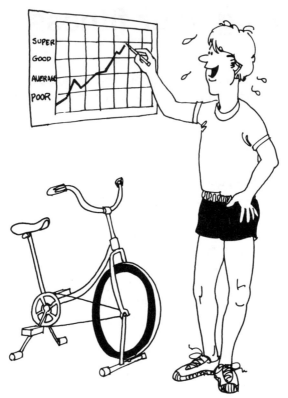

*Self-testing will help you evaluate the effectiveness of your training program.*

However, if used properly, your test results can serve as a highly effective motivational device. The classification charts presented in this chapter for the various tests can show your strengths and weaknesses. Comparing your test results with the charts will give you insight into your physical capabilities. In addition, it will help you evaluate the effectiveness of your training program, be it jogging, swimming, or weight training. Consequently, don't be so concerned with what others can do or cannot do. Self-testing, which is the intent of all the tests in this chapter, will help you make comparisons against yourself. Fitness is individual, so measure your own improvement and watch your progress. If you are careful with your testing procedures, you will know whether you are in shape or out of shape.

Finally, if you are in doubt about your state of health, you are advised to undergo a medical exam before attempting any of these vigorous tests.

This is very important for persons over 30, especially for anyone who has not recently been physically active.

## PHYSICAL FITNESS TEST BATTERY

The specific tests selected for assessing your physical fitness status have all been used successfully in recent years to measure the basic components of physical fitness. They were selected because they provide for uniformity of scoring, consistent measuring, and overall ease in administering. Also minimal time and equipment are required to perform these tests.

The recommended tests for the basic physical fitness components have been grouped into the following areas: (1) muscular strength and endurance, (2) flexibility, and (3) cardiorespiratory endurance. Tests of motor skill performance are also presented for people who wish to evaluate this trait. In addition, a section on evaluating relative body fat is included. The material from this section should be incorporated into your testing program after you read Chapter 9, "Nutrition, Weight Control, and Exercise." For a complete evaluation, a testing program must proceed to measure these traits quantitatively. A reasonable success in all of these tests seems necessary if one is to be classified as physically fit.

The rationale for the tests and instructions for carrying out each test are presented in the separate sections that follow. For women, the step test has been modified to 24 steps per minute, the sit-up test shortened to one minute, and the modified pull-up test is recommended as an alternative to the pull-up test used predominantly by men. The procedures for the remaining tests are the same for men and women.

## INTERPRETING YOUR RESULTS

In each section you will find tables that represent test results of young adult men and women who have been involved in physical conditioning programs in recent years. These composite scores provide a scale on which you can rate your own performances. As mentioned earlier, these norm tables have limitations, because of the problems of interpreting and equating the results for all body types and ages. Nevertheless, although these scales cannot give exact values of your strengths and weaknesses, they can give you a rough indication of them. If you are low in all tests or only in one or two, consider the reasons why, and maybe you can do something about it.

## Interpretation of the Classification Tables

In order to interpret the fitness classification tables (see Tables 3.1 to 3.8) a further explanation is needed. The left-hand margin of each table indicates classifications from "super" down to "very poor." Because it is not statistically permissible to compare or average raw scores from different tests, the scores are all converted to similar units called standard scores. In the tables, the raw scores have been converted to T-scores. This form of standard score ranges from a high score of 80 down to a low score of 20. A T-score of 50 is the mean (average) score for each test and each 10 T-scores is equal to one standard deviation.[1] By converting all your test scores to the same units, you can sum the standard scores for each test and average them to give an overall achievement score for the tests used. For example, an overall average T-score of 57.5 would place you in a very respectable category of "good." This score should not be confused with percentiles. Percentiles cannot be averaged, because they take into account only your position in a group; the actual size of your scores is not considered. The percentile equivalents within the standard deviation units are variable and not comparable. For people who desire to relate the standard scores to percentiles, the table on page 51 provides a comparison, assuming there is a normal distribution of scores. Note, for example, that a T-score of 57.5 (good category) is equivalent to a percentile rank of 77.

## Rating Your Physical Fitness

Physical fitness profile charts can be found at the end of this chapter and in the appendix. Solid lines identify these sheets in the appendix. They can be removed from the book and used in a class situation. They have been constructed to provide flexibility in evaluating your own physical fitness. Use all test items or part of them, such as the three-item series (sit-ups, pull-ups, and distance run) for establishing your physical fitness status. Adding the dodge run and the vertical jump (motor skill performance) to the three-item test gives a broader physical performance rating. Beginning on page 324 of the appendix, conversion tables for changing the raw scores to

---

[1]A standard deviation is a measure of variability that indicates the scatter or spread of approximately two-thirds of a distribution of scores around a mean. When it is used to change test scores into like units (T-scores), you are able to interpret and compare your raw scores from various tests in terms of its position in a normal distribution. For example, a T-score of 60 is one standard deviation above the mean; whereas a T-score of 45 is one-half a standard deviation below the mean. Standard scores provide a simple way to describe the deviation of a test result from the average score for the particular test. These points of reference enable you to judge your position in comparison with others. Your T-score essentially tells you how many standard deviation units you are from the mean.

| T-SCORES | PERCENTILE RANK |
|----------|-----------------|
| 80 | 99.9 |
| 77.5 | 99.7 |
| 75 | 99.4 |
| 72.5 | 98.8 |
| 70 | 97.7 |
| 68.5 | 96.0 |
| 65 | 93.3 |
| 62.5 | 89.4 |
| 60 | 84.1 |
| 57.5 | 77.3 |
| 55 | 69.1 |
| 52.5 | 59.9 |
| 50 | 50 |
| 47.5 | 40.1 |
| 45 | 30.9 |
| 42.5 | 22.7 |
| 40 | 15.9 |
| 37.5 | 10.6 |
| 35.0 | 6.7 |
| 32.5 | 4.0 |
| 30 | 2.3 |
| 27.5 | 1.2 |
| 25.0 | 0.6 |
| 22.5 | 0.3 |
| 20 | 0.1 |

standard scores (T-scores) are given. These charts represent the same values found in the classification tables of this chapter (Tables 3.1 to 3.8), but they are presented in greater detail.

## EVALUATING MUSCULAR STRENGTH AND ENDURANCE

Two fundamental components of physical fitness are muscular strength and muscular endurance. Strength tests have been used as a measure of physical fitness for years. Indeed, the relationship between muscular strength and overall physical condition is quite high. Nevertheless, tests of muscular strength and muscular endurance do not indicate cardiorespiratory endurance, flexibility, and overall athletic ability.

The evaluation procedures recommended here will help you to assess your functional strength and muscular endurance. You can determine whether your strength and endurance are adequate for everyday living and for enjoying your leisure-time activities.

These tests have been used extensively for years and provide reasonable estimates of overall body strength and endurance. Each test has been selected to measure the muscle groups used primarily in moving the weight of the body. The bent-knee sit-ups test the strength and endurance of the abdominal muscles; the pull-ups and dips test the same capacities of the arm and shoulder muscles. The dominant grip test indicates strength. Other criteria that influenced these selections were the ease with which these tests can be scored, the simplicity of administering them, and the high possibility of gaining reliable measurements.

## SIT-UPS* (BENT KNEE)

Purpose: To determine the strength and endurance of the abdominal muscles.

Explanation: Assume a supine position with hands interlocked behind your neck. Draw your feet back toward the buttocks until they are flat on the floor (knees bent). The angle of your legs to your thighs should be approximately 90°. A partner should kneel on one knee, placing it between your feet while grasping both your ankles. A full sit-up is counted when you have curled your back and raised your trunk until your *lower back* is at least perpendicular to the floor and then returned to the starting position. Repeat this procedure as many times as possible within the time limit. The holder counts out loud, emphasizing every fifth sit-up. This assists the performer and also lessens the risk of losing count. The score is the number of sit-ups completed in the selected time period. Resting is permitted, but only on your back with hands in the proper position.

Improper Procedures:  a.  Not coming all the way up to the vertical position. (Do not let your elbows touch your knees—your elbows should pass your knees.)

b.  Releasing your hands from behind your neck. (Do not count these.)

*One minute for women; two minutes for men.

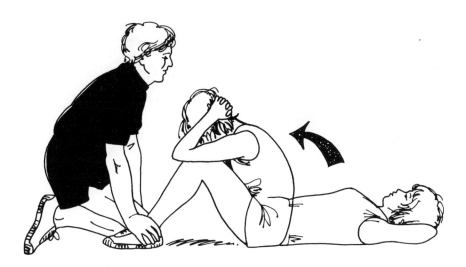

*Sit-up*

**PULL-UP***

| | |
|---|---|
| Purpose: | To test the strength and muscular endurance of the flexors of the arms, shoulder girdle, and upper back muscles. |
| Explanation: | Jump, grasp the overhead bar (palms facing away), and let your legs hang with arms fully extended. Pull up until your chin clears the top of the bar. Then lower yourself to a position of *arms fully extended.* Repeat this procedure until you can no longer continue.<br>In scoring, record only the complete chins. |

Improper Procedures.
    a.   Legs swinging or kicking.
    b.   Failure to return to a "dead hang" (elbows straight; this is *a must* for the exercise to be valid.)
    c.   Failure of the chin to rise above the bar.

*Although no values for women are presented in the tables, they can safely perform this exercise.

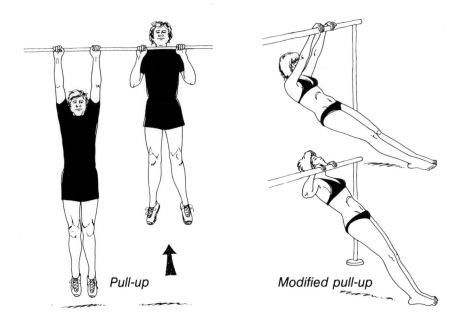

*Pull-up*    *Modified pull-up*

## MODIFIED PULL-UP*

Purpose:     To test the strength and muscular endurance of the flexors of the arms, shoulder girdle, and upper back muscles.

Explanation: An adjustable horizontal bar should be set at approximately the height of the apex of your sternum (breastbone). Grasp the bar, palms outward. Slide feet under the bar until your body and extended arms form a right angle. Your body should be held in a firm straight position, with your weight on the rear of your feet. A partner should kneel on one knee, placing it between your feet while supporting your ankles. Now begin from this extended body and arm position and pull your chest to the bar. Repeat as many times as possible, keeping your body straight.

In scoring record only properly performed pull-ups.

Improper Procedures:   a.   Body sags.
                       b.   Hips rise (hip motion).
                       c.   Failure to complete pull-up.

---

*This test can be used for people who are unable to do a complete pull-up on an overhead bar. Women are ordinarily tested this way; however, this test can be used for men who are very weak in the upper body or who are very obese.

## DIPS

Purpose: To test the strength and muscle endurance of the extensors of the arms, shoulder girdle, and upper back muscles.

Explanation: You start from an arm rest position at the end of parallel bars, with arms fully extended. From this position, lower your body to a right-angle arm-bend position. Then you push (extend arms) to the starting position. Scoring consists of recording only the complete dips.

Improper Procedures:
    a. Swinging or kicking up into a dip.
    b. Partial dips. (You must lower yourself all the way down so that your upper arm is parallel to the horizontal.)

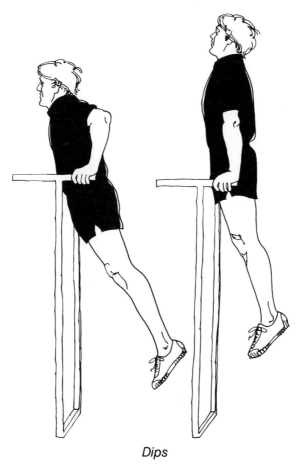

*Dips*

## GRIP STRENGTH (DOMINANT HAND)

Purpose: To test the strength of muscles of the fingers, hand, and forearm.

Explanation: Using a grip dynamometer, adjust it so that it fits your dominant hand comfortably. Then squeeze the dynamometer

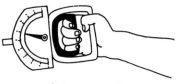

*Grip strength*

## TABLE 3.1. MUSCULAR STRENGTH AND ENDURANCE (WOMEN)

| | T-SCORE | DOMINANT GRIP (Kg.) | ONE MINUTE SIT-UPS (No.) | MODIFIED PULL-UPS (No.) |
|---|---|---|---|---|
| | 80.0 | 45.0 | 45 | 41 |
| Super | 75.0 | 42.5 | 41 | 37 |
| | 70.0 | 40.0 | 38 | 34 |
| | 67.5 | 39.0 | 37 | 32 |
| Excellent | 65.0 | 37.5 | 35 | 30 |
| | 62.5 | 36.5 | 33 | 29 |
| | 60.0 | 35.0 | 31 | 27 |
| Good | 57.5 | 34.0 | 29 | 25 |
| | 55.0 | 32.5 | 28 | 23 |
| | 52.5 | 31.5 | 26 | 22 |
| Average | 50.0 | 30.0 | 24 | 20 |
| | 47.5 | 29.0 | 23 | 18 |
| | 45.0 | 27.5 | 21 | 16 |
| Fair | 42.5 | 26.5 | 19 | 15 |
| | 40.0 | 25.0 | 17 | 13 |
| | 37.5 | 24.0 | 15 | 11 |
| Poor | 35.0 | 22.5 | 14 | 9 |
| | 32.5 | 21.5 | 12 | 8 |
| | 30.0 | 20.0 | 10 | 6 |
| Very poor | 25.0 | 17.5 | 6 | 3 |
| | 20.0 | 15.0 | 3 | 0 |

vigorously. A downward thrust is allowed. Repeat the test and record your best score, as read from the dial, in kilograms.

Improper Procedures: Do not allow your hand, arm, or elbow to touch the body or any object while performing the test.

## FLEXIBILITY EVALUATION

Flexibility is the ability to use a muscle throughout its maximum range of motion. The loss of the ability to bend, twist, and stretch is a result of muscle disuse, such as in excessive periods of sitting or standing. Sedentary living habits can lead to shortened muscles and tendons, low back pain, and an imbalance of strength between opposing pairs of muscles. The shortening of the hamstrings (muscles located in the back of the thighs) is a very common disorder. Long periods of sitting or standing lead

## TABLE 3.2. MUSCULAR STRENGTH AND ENDURANCE (MEN)

|  | T-SCORE | DOMINANT GRIP (Kg.) | TWO-MINUTE SIT-UPS (No.) | PULL-UPS (No.) | DIPS (No.) |
|---|---|---|---|---|---|
| Super | 80.0 | 73.0 | 91 | 19 | 28 |
|  | 75.0 | 69.5 | 85 | 17 | 25 |
|  | 70.0 | 65.5 | 79 | 15 | 23 |
| Excellent | 67.5 | 64.0 | 76 | 14 | 22 |
|  | 65.0 | 62.0 | 73 | 13 | 20 |
|  | 62.5 | 60.0 | 69 | 12 | 19 |
| Good | 60.0 | 58.5 | 67 | 11 | 18 |
|  | 57.5 | 56.5 | 65 | 10 | 17 |
|  | 55.0 | 55.0 | 62 | 9 | 15 |
| Average | 52.5 | 53.0 | 59 | 8 | 14 |
|  | 50.0 | 51.0 | 56 | 7 | 13 |
|  | 47.5 | 48.5 | 52 | 6 | 11 |
| Fair | 45.0 | 48.0 | 50 | 5 | 9 |
|  | 42.5 | 45.5 | 47 | 4 | 8 |
|  | 40.0 | 44.0 | 44 | 3 | 7 |
| Poor | 37.5 | 42.0 | 41 | 2 | 6 |
|  | 35.0 | 40.0 | 38 | 1 | 4 |
|  | 32.5 | 38.0 | 35 | 0 | 3 |
| Very poor | 30.0 | 36.5 | 32 | 0 | 2 |
|  | 25.0 | 33.0 | 26 | 0 | 0 |
|  | 20.0 | 29.0 | 21 | 0 | 0 |

to poor muscle and tendon adjustments and a loss of flexibility in these muscles. This loss of flexibility limits your ability to walk smoothly, to sit down or stand up gracefully, and to perform efficiently in recreational pursuits. Extreme flexibility, however, has no advantage. If your joints are too loose or flexible, you may become more susceptible to injuries of the joints. It is much more normal to be able to stretch one or two inches (plus or minus) from the mean. In other words, too much flexibility may increase the chance of injury. Exercises for stretching the major muscle groups are recommended in Chapter 5, "Individualized Conditioning Exercises." Although no single test will provide adequate information about the flexibility of all the major joints of the body, the following two tests provide a reasonable indication of your ability to stretch.

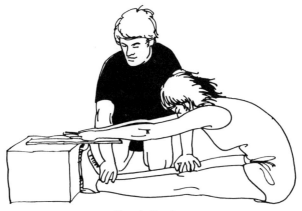

*Trunk flexion*

## TRUNK FLEXION

Purpose:      To measure the amount of trunk flexion and the ability to stretch the back muscles and back thigh muscles (hamstrings).

Explanation:  Sit with your legs fully extended and the bottom of your feet flat against a board projecting from the wall. Now extend (stretch) your arms and hands forward as far as possible and hold for a count of three. With a ruler, measure (in inches) the distance before or beyond the edge of the board that you reach. Distances before the edge (not able to reach your toes) are expressed as negative scores; those beyond the edge are expressed as positive scores.

Improper Procedures:  a.  Not holding the flexed position for a count of three.
                       b.  Bending at the knees.

NORMS FOR TRUNK FLEXION

|  | WOMEN | MEN |
|---|---|---|
| Normal range | +4 to +10 in. | -6 to +8 in. |
| Average (mean) | +2 in. | +1 in. |
| Desired range | +2 to +6 in. | +1 to +5 in. |

## TRUNK EXTENSION

Purpose:  To measure the range of motion (flexibility) of the back.

Explanation:  Lie in a prone position (face down) on the floor. Have a partner kneel and straddle your legs, holding your buttocks and legs down. With your hands grasped behind your neck,

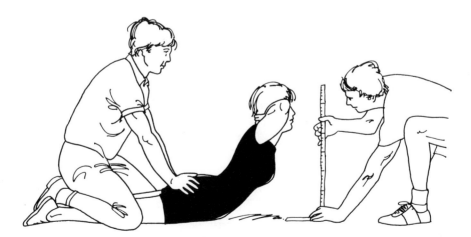

*Trunk extension*

raise your upper trunk (chest and head) off the floor and hold for a count of three. Measure the distance from your chin to the floor.

Improper Procedures:   a.  Not holding the measuring device in a perpendicular position while measuring.
                          b.  Raising the hips off the floor.
                          c.  Not holding the extended position for a count of three.

NORMS FOR TRUNK EXTENSION

|  | WOMEN | MEN |
|---|---|---|
| Normal range | 12 to 30 in. | 4 to 27 in. |
| Average (mean) | 21 in. | 15 in. |
| Desired range | 21 to 25 in. | 15 to 20 in. |

## MOTOR SKILL EVALUATION

General motor skill has been defined as one's level of ability in a wide range of physical activities. Speed, power, balance, agility, reaction time, and coordination are the traits identified with motor skill performance. In successful performance, these skills blend into an effective movement, such as stroking a tennis ball. A movement may be quite complex. For example, hitting a forehand in tennis involves three moving factors: the ball, the body (feet), and the racquet. Integration of motor abilities in a coordinated manner leads to graceful movement.

The skills involved in each sport are quite specific. Success in one activity does not necessarily mean equal success in another. It is impossible to measure all the specifics of complex physical activities. An acceptable alternative has been to sample some of the specific traits involved in athletic performance to gain insight into one's general motor ability. A person who scores well on a motor skill test usually has the potential for successful performance in a sport making use of this skill after instruction and practice. Tests of motor ability may reflect a person's potential in specific sports skills.

The tests recommended here do not examine all the traits related to general motor ability. However, the vertical jump, agility run, and squat thrusts have emerged as excellent indicators of general athletic ability. Again based on the criteria of time taken to perform these tests, the ease in administering and in scoring them, these tests are practical tools for testing general motor skill performance.

## AGILITY RUN (ILLINOIS)

Purpose: To measure your ability to move with quickness, speed, and balance.

Explanation: Start in a front lying position behind the starting line with your arms flexed and hands placed just outside your shoulder. On the command "go" the stop watch starts, jump to your feet and run as fast as you can to the end line, a

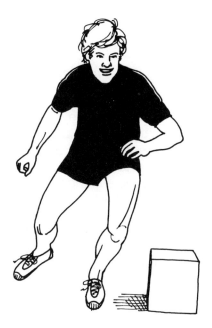

*Agility run*

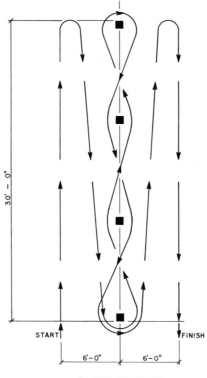

30' – 0"

START ↑     ↓ FINISH

6'–0"     6'–0"

ILLINOIS AGILITY RUN

*Diagram for agility run*

distance of 30 feet (see diagram); stop as one foot touches or crosses the end line and then sprint back to starting line. Then weave in and out around four chairs spaced 10 feet apart to the end line, and then turn and weave back through the chairs to the starting line. You then sprint to the end line, touch or cross it with your foot, and turn and sprint past the finish line. The time necessary to complete the run is recorded to the nearest tenth of a second. A wet towel may be provided so you can wipe off your feet before the run. This allows better traction during the run.

Improper Procedures:   a.   Not touching the lines at each end.
                                 b.   Touching or accidently touching the chair.
                                 c.   Not following the prescribed course.

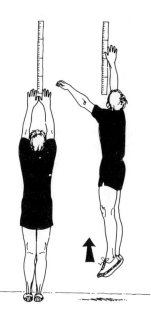

*Vertical jump*

## VERTICAL JUMP

Purpose: To test the power of the extensor muscles of the hips, knees, and ankles.

Explanation: Face the jumping board and stand slightly in front of it, with your feet flat on the floor and both arms fully extended overhead. Note the point where the extended tips of the middle fingers touch the board. Now turn, so that a side of your body is to the jumpboard. Without moving your feet (you are not allowed a step into the jump), take a deep squat and jump, touching the board as high as possible with the fingers nearest the board. After a brief rest, try a second jump. Record the greatest distance obtained between your standing reach and your jumping reach, to the nearest half-inch.

Improper Procedures:  a.  Not getting a true standing reach.
                      b.  Moving the feet in preparation to jump.

## SQUAT THRUSTS

| | |
|---|---|
| Purpose: | To determine your ability to move large muscle groups rapidly and to sustain this total body movement for a specific period of time. |
| Explanation: | Stand erect with feet together and hands at your sides. This is a four-count exercise. (1) Assume a position with hands on the floor in front of your feet with knees bent. (2) Then thrust your legs back to an extended position (a front support position). (3) Quickly bring your legs back to the squat position. (4) Then straighten to a standing position. This represents one complete repetition. Your score is determined by the number of complete and partial repetitions you can perform in 30 seconds. For example, if you complete 15 reps and are in the squat position prior to standing at the end of 30 seconds, you would score 15-3. |

Improper Procedures:   a.   Not coming to the squat position before extending out to the front support position.

                       b.   Not returning to the squat position before standing.

                       c.   Not standing erect at the end of each rep.

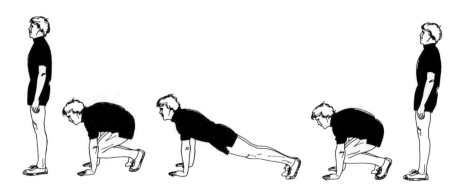

*Squat thrusts*

# EVALUATING YOUR CARDIORESPIRATORY ENDURANCE

As we saw in Chapter 2, the ability of the heart to pump blood, of the lungs to breathe volumes of air, and of the muscles to utilize oxygen are measures of the quality of one's cardiorespiratory fitness. Sustained muscular activity is possible only through the effective functioning of the heart, blood vessels, and lungs. Tests involving vigorous physical movement that make increased demands on the heart and lungs have been devised as sound measures of cardiorespiratory endurance and health.

Some of these tests will be presented here. From this selection, which includes running tests, a heart-rate recovery test, and a simple exercise heart-rate test on a stationary bike, you ought to be able to find one or two of these measures that will help you gain some insight into your cardiorespiratory fitness.

## TABLE 3.3  MOTOR SKILL PERFORMANCE (WOMEN)

|           | T-SCORE | VERTICAL JUMP (in.) | AGILITY RUN (sec) | SQUAT THRUSTS (no. in 30 sec) |
|-----------|---------|---------------------|-------------------|-------------------------------|
|           | 80.0    | 20.0                | 15.9              | 19                            |
| Super     | 75.0    | 18.5                | 16.8              | 18                            |
|           | 70.0    | 17.5                | 17.7              | 17                            |
|           | 67.5    | 17.0                | 18.1              | 16-2                          |
| Excellent | 65.0    | 16.5                | 18.6              | 16                            |
|           | 62.5    | 16.0                | 19.0              | 15-2                          |
|           | 60.0    | 15.0                | 19.5              | 15                            |
| Good      | 57.5    | 14.5                | 19.9              | 14-2                          |
|           | 55.0    | 14.0                | 20.4              | 14                            |
|           | 52.5    | 13.5                | 20.8              | 13-2                          |
| Average   | 50.0    | 13.0                | 21.3              | 13                            |
|           | 47.5    | 12.5                | 21.7              | 12-2                          |
|           | 45.0    | 12.0                | 22.2              | 12                            |
| Fair      | 42.5    | 11.5                | 22.6              | 11-2                          |
|           | 40.0    | 11.0                | 23.1              | 11                            |
|           | 37.5    | 10.5                | 23.5              | 10-2                          |
| Poor      | 35.0    | 10.0                | 24.0              | 10                            |
|           | 32.5    | 9.0                 | 24.4              | 9-2                           |
|           | 30.0    | 8.5                 | 24.9              | 9                             |
| Very poor | 25.0    | 7.5                 | 25.8              | 8                             |
|           | 20.0    | 6.5                 | 26.7              | 7                             |

## TABLE 3.4    MOTOR SKILL PERFORMANCE (MEN)

|  | T-SCORE | VERTICAL JUMP (in.) | AGILITY RUN (sec) | SQUAT THRUSTS (no. in 30 sec) |
|---|---|---|---|---|
| Super | 80.0 | 27.5 | 15.3 | 23 |
|  | 75.0 | 26.5 | 15.7 | 22 |
|  | 70.0 | 25.5 | 16.1 | 21 |
| Excellent | 67.5 | 25.0 | 16.3 | 20-2 |
|  | 65.0 | 24.5 | 16.5 | 20 |
|  | 62.5 | 24.0 | 16.7 | 19-2 |
| Good | 60.0 | 23.5 | 16.9 | 19 |
|  | 57.5 | 23.0 | 17.1 | 18-2 |
|  | 55.0 | 22.5 | 17.3 | 18 |
| Average | 52.5 | 22.0 | 17.5 | 17-2 |
|  | 50.0 | 21.5 | 17.7 | 17 |
|  | 47.5 | 21.0 | 17.9 | 16-2 |
| Fair | 45.0 | 20.5 | 18.1 | 16 |
|  | 42.5 | 20.0 | 18.3 | 15-2 |
|  | 40.0 | 19.5 | 18.5 | 15 |
| Poor | 37.5 | 19.0 | 18.7 | 14-2 |
|  | 35.0 | 18.5 | 18.9 | 14 |
|  | 32.5 | 18.0 | 19.1 | 13-2 |
| Very poor | 30.0 | 17.5 | 19.3 | 13 |
|  | 25.0 | 16.5 | 19.7 | 12 |
|  | 20.0 | 15.5 | 20.1 | 11 |

## Aerobic Capacity Field Tests

Procedures for determining aerobic capacity in the laboratory are complex, time-consuming, and impractical for determining cardiorespiratory fitness levels in large numbers of people. Recent studies, therefore, have attempted to develop field tests that can be substituted for laboratory tests. Field tests, such as a two-mile or 12-minute run have correlated well with laboratory-determined values for physiological factors such as maximal oxygen uptake. Thus these types of tests provide results in understandable terms, making it easy to determine your own physical fitness and to perceive changes due to training. Most field tests of cardiorespiratory endurance utilize running, jogging, or walking. Studies have aimed at determining how long a person must work to provide accurate results. Dr. Bruno

Balke, a physiologist, has demonstrated that an adequate estimate of your aerobic capacity is possible after as little as 10 minutes of maximal work. Other studies confirm that the duration of a running test must be between 10 and 20 minutes to provide reasonable estimates of aerobic capacity. This is because if shorter runs, such as 600 yards or even a mile, are completed in less than 8 to 10 minutes much of the energy used comes from anaerobic energy sources. (See Chapter 2 for a more detailed explanation of anaerobic metabolism.) Figure 3.1 shows the relative roles of anaerobic and aerobic energy for intervals of work of up to 15 minutes. The graph demonstrates that during a "best-effort" one-minute run, slightly more than 60 % of the work is performed anaerobically. (This means that 60% of the total energy requirements is derived *without* oxygen; instead it is derived from the splitting of energy-rich substances stored within the muscles.) As the duration of a "best-effort" run increases, the demand on the anaerobic energy component is less, and it decreases to less than 10 percent after 10 minutes. The significant point is that if maximum work is

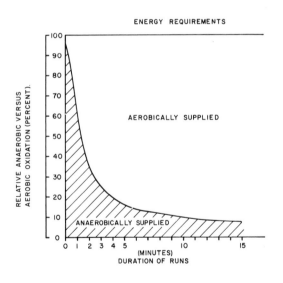

*Figure 3.1*

The relative role of anaerobic and aerobic oxidation for supplying amounts of oxygen required during best-effort runs of defined time intervals.
(Redrawn from Balke, Bruno, "A Simple Field Test For The Assessment of Physical Fitness"—U.S. Government Printing Office, 1963.

performed for 10 to 20 minutes, the predominant energy source is dependent on the utilization of oxygen; thus an adequate estimate of one's aerobic capacity will result. Consequently, the 12-minute run or 1½ to 2-mile run have proved to be effective indicators of cardiorespiratory fitness.

Dr. Ken Cooper, of the Institute for Aerobics Research of Dallas, has applied the original work of Balke and developed a 12-minute run test for estimating maximal oxygen uptake. The runner is to cover as much distance as possible in 12 minutes. The distance covered is generally recorded to the nearest ⅛ mile (220 yards). In men the correlation between Cooper's test and the aerobic capacity determined on a laboratory treadmill was 0.90, a very high relationship. For women, however, the correlation has not been as high. Dr. Paul Ribisl, a physical fitness researcher at Wake Forest University, has shown a similarly high relationship between the two-mile run and laboratory tests. Both these results support Balke's requirement of a minimum duration of 10 minutes. Actually, Balke found 15 minutes to be the optimum duration for estimating aerobic capacity.

Our own work produced a correlation of 0.88 between the times of men in the two-mile run and their maximal oxygen uptake as measured on a treadmill. For college-aged women joggers, we have correlated the time for 1.5-mile run with maximal oxygen uptake. This produced a 0.91 correlation.

Five fitness classifications are provided (Tables 3.5 and 3.6) to assist you in rating yourself according to the time required to run a 1.5-mile distance (for women) or a 2-mile distance (for men). In addition, because the time to run these distances correlates very well with your maximal oxygen uptake, estimates of your aerobic capacity are given in accordance with your running times.

TABLE 3.5.   CLASSIFICATION OF 1.5-MILE RUN TIMES FOR YOUNG ADULT FEMALES

| FITNESS CATEGORY | 1.5-MILE TIME | ESTIMATED MAXIMAL OXYGEN UPTAKE EQUIVALENTS |
|---|---|---|
| Super | Faster than 11:30 | 50 ml/kg·min or higher |
| Excellent | 11:30 to 12:59 | 49.9 to 44.0 ml/kg·min |
| Good | 13:00 to 14:29 | 43.9 to 38.0 ml/kg·min |
| Fair | 14:30 to 15:59 | 37.9 to 32.0 ml/kg·min |
| Poor | 16:00 or slower | 31.9 ml/kg·min or lower |

## TABLE 3.6.  CLASSIFICATION OF 2-MILE RUN TIMES FOR YOUNG ADULT MALES

| FITNESS CATEGORY | 2-MILE TIME | ESTIMATED MAXIMAL OXYGEN UPTAKE EQUIVALENTS |
|---|---|---|
| Super | Faster than 12:00 | 55 ml/kg·min or higher |
| Excellent | 12:00 to 13:59 | 54.9 to 50 ml/kg·min |
| Good | 14:00 to 15:59 | 49.9 to 45 ml/kg·min |
| Fair | 16:00 to 17:59 | 44.9 to 40 ml/kg·min |
| Poor | 18:00 or slower | 39.9 ml/kg·min or lower |

In addition, Tables 3.7 and 3.8 enable you to compare your cardiorespiratory test results with other young men and women. T-score scales for the 12-minute run, 1-, 1.5- and 2-mile runs are listed along with a scale for the step test *recovery index* score, the topic of the next section.

### A Heart-Rate Recovery Test

Another useful procedure for assessing your cardiorespiratory fitness is the step test a heart-rate recovery measure. Stepping on and off a bench for a three-to-five minute time period at a selected cadence (24 or 30 steps a minute) has long been used for rating the physical capacity for hard work and evaluating the effects of training. Although not recognized as the best

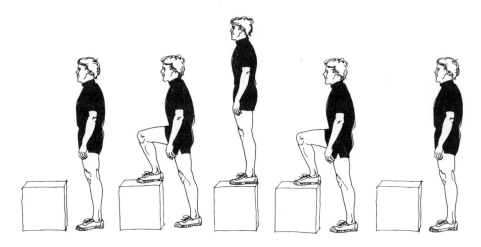

*Figure 3.2    Step test*

predictor of cardiorespiratory fitness, the heart-rate reaction during recovery from a standardized step test is a simple way to evaluate the heart's response to exercise. The test is easy to administer on an individual basis or to a large group. It takes little time, does not require special skills to perform and, more important, requires a minimum of equipment (locker room bench or bleachers, watch, and a card for recording pulse counts). The testing can easily be done with the methods and procedures described here.

### Step-Test Procedure

1. A locker room bench (generally 18 in. high) is recommended for both men and women. A roll-out bleacher seat (usually 16 in. high) can be used. If neither is available, a sturdy chair (17 in. high) can be used. (Step-test norms presented in the T-Score charts are based on stepping up on an 18 in. bench.)

2. Work with a partner.

3. As soon as the signal is given to "begin," the watch is started and you start stepping on to the bench; first the left foot *up,* then the right foot *up.* Then the left foot *down,* then the right foot *down.* (See Figure 3.2). This represents 4 counts. Step in cadence at the following pace:

   Men: 120 counts/minute or 30-step executions/minute (4-step count every 2 seconds—up, up, down, down).

   Women: 96 counts/minute or 24-step executions/minute (4-step count every 2.5 seconds—up, up, down, down).

4. Continue the exercise for 3 minutes. Keep the tempo and be sure to straighten the knees as you step on the bench. (In a group situation, the instructor will keep the cadence.)

5. Measurements

   a. After stepping for 3 minutes, sit on the bench or chair.

   b. One minute after the exercise period stops, the tester counts the pulse for 30 seconds. (In a group situation, the instructor calls out BEGIN and STOP for each 30-second period.)

   c. Record the pulse for the following periods:

      1–1½ minutes of recovery
      2–2½ minutes of recovery
      3–3½ minutes of recovery

6. Measuring the Pulse:
   The tester presses lightly with the index and middle fingers in the region just below the jawbone, and just behind the Adam's apple. For added accuracy the performer can check his pulse also at the radial artery site, located on the inside of the wrist, thumb-side. This measurement provides a double check for accuracy, and the rate should not differ more than two beats from the tester's count during a 30-second period. A stethoscope, if available, provides the best means for accuracy.

7. Improper Procedures:
   a. Not keeping the cadence of 30 or 24 step executions per minute.
   b. Failure to straighten the knees to full extension on the step ups.

8. Scoring:
   The sum of the three 30-second pulses is your <u>recovery index.</u>

   On a three-by-five inch card make a testing card as shown below for recording each recovery pulse. Be sure to mark the time of day and the date. Refer to this when you repeat the step test at a later date.

---

STEP TEST ( _____ min)
Stepping Rate _____
NAME _____ _____ AGE _____
RECOVERIES (beats)
   1-1½ min _____
   2-2½ min _____
   3-3½ min _____
   Total _____
     (Recovery Index)
DATE: _____
TIME: _____     BENCH HEIGHT _____ in.

Compare your personal recovery index for the step test with norms given in the cardiorespiratory Tables 3.7 (women) or 3.8 (men). These tables

## TABLE 3.7.  CARDIORESPIRATORY (WOMEN)

|  | T-SCORE | 1-MILE RUN (min) | 1.5-MILE RUN (min) | 12-MINUTE RUN (220-yd laps) | 3-MINUTE STEP TEST (Recovery Index) |
|---|---|---|---|---|---|
| Super | 80.0 | 5:00 | 9:54 | 13 | 95 |
|  | 75.0 | 5:45 | 10:47 |  | 107 |
|  | 70.0 | 6:30 | 11:40 |  | 118 |
| Excellent | 67.5 | 6:53 | 12:06 | 12 | 126 |
|  | 65.0 | 7:15 | 12:33 |  | 130 |
|  | 62.5 | 7:38 | 13:00 |  | 135 |
| Good | 60.0 | 8:00 | 13:26 | 11 | 141 |
|  | 57.5 | 8:23 | 13:53 |  | 147 |
|  | 55.0 | 8:45 | 14:19 |  | 153 |
| Average | 52.5 | 9:08 | 14:46 | 10 | 158 |
|  | 50.0 | 9:30 | 15:12 |  | 164 |
|  | 47.5 | 9:53 | 15:38 |  | 170 |
| Fair | 45.0 | 10:15 | 16:04 | 9 | 176 |
|  | 42.5 | 10:38 | 16:31 |  | 181 |
|  | 40.0 | 11:00 | 16:57 |  | 187 |
| Poor | 37.5 | 11:23 | 17:24 | 8 | 193 |
|  | 35.0 | 11:45 | 17:50 |  | 199 |
|  | 32.5 | 12:08 | 18:17 |  | 204 |
| Very poor | 30.0 | 12:30 | 18:43 | 7 | 210 |
|  | 25.0 | 13:15 | 19:36 |  | 222 |
|  | 20.0 | 14:00 | 20:29 |  | 233 |

contain the scores for college-aged men and women who performed the test on an 18 inch bench. They will give you some indication of the functional ability of your heart. Use your initial *recovery index* as your starting point. As you continue your physical conditioning program, you can compare your heart-rate recovery rates, that is, check your progress. Basically, you are competing against yourself. Be sure to repeat the test under similar conditions: for example, time of day, temperature, no physical activity prior to test, and so on. As your heart and muscles become better conditioned, your *recovery index* (sum of the three recoveries) will decrease. Recovery indexes falling below 150 are good scores. Highly trained individuals tend to score below 120, which indicates an excellent response of the cardiorespiratory system.

# TABLE 3.8. CARDIORESPIRATORY (MEN)

|  | T-SCORE | 1-MILE RUN (min) | 2-MILE RUN (min) | 12-MINUTE RUN (220 yd laps) | 3-MINUTE STEP TEST (Recovery Index) |
|---|---|---|---|---|---|
| | 80.0 | 4:15 | 10:14 | 18.0 | 97 |
| Super | 75.0 | 4:38 | 10:59 | 17.5 | 107 |
| | 70.0 | 5:00 | 11:44 | 17.0 | 117 |
| | 67.5 | 5:11 | 12:07 | 16.5 | 122 |
| Excellent | 65.0 | 5:23 | 12:29 | 16.0 | 127 |
| | 62.5 | 5:34 | 12:52 | 15.5 | 132 |
| | 60.0 | 5:45 | 13:14 | 15.0 | 137 |
| Good | 57.5 | 5:56 | 13:37 | 14.5 | 142 |
| | 55.0 | 6:08 | 13:59 | 14.0 | 147 |
| | 52.5 | 6:19 | 14:22 | 13.5 | 152 |
| Average | 50.0 | 6:30 | 14:46 | 13.0 | 157 |
| | 47.5 | 6:41 | 15:09 | 12.5 | 162 |
| | 45.0 | 6:53 | 15:31 | 12.0 | 167 |
| Fair | 42.5 | 7:04 | 15:54 | 11.5 | 172 |
| | 40.0 | 7:15 | 16:16 | 11.0 | 177 |
| | 37.5 | 7:26 | 16:39 | 10.5 | 182 |
| Poor | 35.0 | 7:38 | 17:01 | 10.0 | 187 |
| | 32.5 | 7:49 | 17:24 | 9.5 | 192 |
| | 30.0 | 8:00 | 17:46 | 9.0 | 197 |
| Very poor | 25.0 | 8:23 | 18:31 | 8.5 | 207 |
| | 20.0 | 8:45 | 19:16 | 8.0 | 217 |

Our experience has shown that the step test has encouraged an increased awareness and understanding about physical fitness in participants. You can read all you want about the heart rate during exercise and recovery, but nothing demonstrates the phenomenon more effectively than actually observing the responses of your own heart rate to exercise.

## An Exercise Heart-Rate Test
In Chapter 6 we make suggestions for a physical conditioning program using the stationary bicycle (often called a bicycle ergometer). Access to such a device for training is limited. However some colleges, YM/YWCA's, and health clubs are now providing exercise ergometers in their exercise rooms. With this possibility in mind, a simple bike test for following the

progress of your cardiorespiratory training program will be presented. Recall (Chapter 2) that heart-rate responses to standardized work loads can serve as convenient indicators of physical fitness capacities and changes. The bicycle ergometer provides an accurate measurement of the work performed. It can be adjusted so that the person pedaling can experience a graded and measurable work load. The pedaling of the bike during a prolonged period puts a demand on the heart and related circulatory functions. The physiological adjustment to a given work load gives a fair indication of one's capacity to exercise. Determining your heart rate during selected segments of graded work is a good way to judge your physical fitness capacity. The more highly fit you are, the lower the heart rate for a given work load.

### *Procedure for Self-Testing*

Besides the ergometer, all you need is a watch with a second hand (a wall clock is all right) and someone to check your heart rate as you exercise. (See page 71 for ways to measure the heart rate.) A stethoscope, if available, will assure more accuracy in measuring the heart beats during the pedaling exercise. You need to adjust the saddle and handlebar to a comfortable position. To get the proper saddle height you must have the front part of your foot on the pedal (in the lower position) with the knee joint slightly bent.

Each manufacturer has a work load setting, with the rate of work usually expressed in watts or kilogram-meters. Generally, the first work load should be very light—a warm-up. For example, on the Monark Bicycle or the Schwinn Ergo-Metric Exerciser a load setting of 1.0 is a suitable beginning point. This is equivalent to almost 5 Calories of energy, or 300 kilogram-meters. This load equals 50 watts on an electric bike. Your pedaling rate should be 60 turns per minute.

Begin pedaling, noting the time. After about a minute of pedaling, check your pulse or heart rate for 15 seconds and multiply by four to get your heart beats per minute (bpm). After 4 to 5 minutes your heart rate will reach a steady state, that is, level off. If the difference between these heart rates (fourth and fifth minutes) exceeds 8 beats, then the working time should be continued for one or more minutes more until a constant level is reached. The average for the last two measured heart rates represents your exercising heart rate for that work load.

After recording your heart rate for the initial bout of work, set the load at a heavier level and repeat the test (Table 3.9). The second work load should

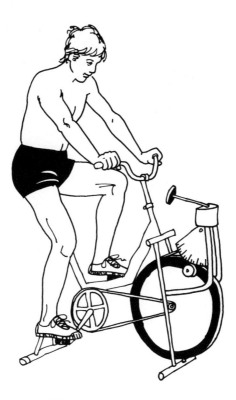

*Bicycle ergometer test*

## TABLE 3.9.   SUGGESTED FORM FOR RECORDING YOUR HEART-RATE RESPONSE DURING THE ERGOMETER TEST

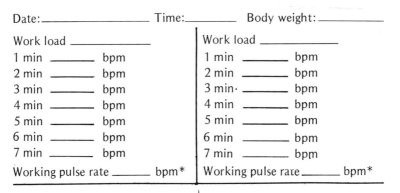

Date:_____ Time:_____ Body weight:_____

| Work load _____ | Work load _____ |
| --- | --- |
| 1 min _____ bpm | 1 min _____ bpm |
| 2 min _____ bpm | 2 min _____ bpm |
| 3 min _____ bpm | 3 min· _____ bpm |
| 4 min _____ bpm | 4 min _____ bpm |
| 5 min _____ bpm | 5 min _____ bpm |
| 6 min _____ bpm | 6 min _____ bpm |
| 7 min _____ bpm | 7 min _____ bpm |
| Working pulse rate _____ bpm* | Working pulse rate _____ bpm* |

*The mean of the final two heart rates (beats per min).

be heavy enough to illicit a heart rate of 140 beats per minute or higher. As a guide, if your first bout of work required a heart rate under 100, triple your load; if your heart rate is under 120, increase the work load by 2.5; if your heart rate is over 120, then double the work load.

This simple heart-rate test, if repeated at different periods of your training program (such as every five weeks), will enable you to follow your progress and improvement quite easily. By repeating the exact procedures each time, you can determine objectively the effects of your training on your circulatory system. Effective training will be accompanied by a lower heart rate for the selected work load. Figure 3.3 shows the training effects of the heart's response to a standard work load (900 kilogram-meters or a setting of "3" on the Monark or Schwinn Bike) throughout a 20-week program of jogging. According to research studies this decrease in the heart rate during exercise results from improved <u>stroke volume</u> of the heart and an improved efficiency of the cardiorespiratory systems.

Many variations of bicycle ergometer tests have been devised. Some of them estimate one's maximal oxygen uptake based on heart-rate responses to submaximal work loads. Estimating one's aerobic capacity in

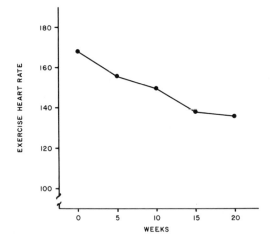

*Figure 3.3 Heart rate during steady state work on a bicycle ergometer throughout a 20 week training period. Work load equivalent to: 3 setting (Schwinn Ergometric), 150 watts, 900 kpm (Monark)*

this manner has been widely criticized, and errors of prediction can be quite large. Nevertheless, submaximal effort tests of this kind can roughly reflect the cardiorespiratory endurance of an individual. This knowledge can be wisely used for planning an exercise program that suits an individual's needs. You can easily make your own chart and plot your progress over the weeks of training.

The following three sources are recommended for obtaining detailed methods and tables for predicting maximal oxygen uptake from submaximal heart-rate measurements on a bicycle ergometer.

Astrand, Per-Olof and Kaare Rodahl, *Textbooks of Work Physiology.* New York: McGraw-Hill, 1970, pages 349–362, 617–620.

deVries, Herbert A., *Laboratory Experiments in Physiology of Exercise.* Dubuque, Iowa: W. C. Brown, 1971, pages 83–94.

National Council of YMCAs, *The Y's Way to Physical Fitness.* Myers, Clayton, Lawrence Golding and Wayne Sinning, eds. Emmaus, Pa.: Rodale Press, 1973.

## ANALYSIS OF BODY FAT AND BODY BUILD

The importance of establishing good nutritional and exercise habits for enhancing the natural proportions of your body is emphasized in Chapter 9. This section is intended to help you gain information about your body proportions and to determine a desirable weight for you. Measurements of selected girths and fat skinfolds can be useful in setting personal weight control goals.

The sex of a person and one's genetic background determine the distribution of fat deposits on the body. Men and women do not put on fat (or lose it) in the same places. In addition, we do know that fatness runs in families. But we don't know how much of this tendency to be fat is inherited or a result of eating habits formed in the home. Exercise can be an important means for controlling your body fat and overall body build. Furthermore, a well-balanced body shape reflects self-confidence and pride. Exercise helps to give your muscles pleasing shapes and contours, and muscles are what give shape to your body. In addition, exercise can redistribute your weight by toning up muscles (making them firmer) and by aiding you in losing excess fat.

Here are some techniques for measuring your body fat, your body girths, and determining a desired weight.

## Body Fat Evaluation

Being overweight due to a preponderance of bone and muscle does not have the same meaning as being overweight due to fat tissue. Quite often, an improvement in physical fitness is accompanied by a reduction in body fat. Even when exercise does not result in the loss of weight the amount of body fat may be reduced. This is because the relative proportions of <u>lean body weight</u> and fat change. The stored fat in the body is reduced, and the lean body weight (primarily muscles) is increased.

Body fat and lean body weight can be measured quite accurately in the laboratory. However, because of the elaborate equipment, complex procedures, and substantial time required to test each invidual, these methods are not widely used. As a result, researchers have developed other means for estimating body fat that are closely related to the complex laboratory techniques. Fortunately, simple methods using <u>skinfold calipers</u> are quite suitable for determining lean body weight and <u>fat weight.</u>

Dr. A. W. Sloan and his fellow researchers have developed formulas for estimating <u>body density</u> using two skinfold measurements as predictors. For young men, the fat thickness at the subscapula and thigh sites have proven to be a good gauge of overall body fatness. For young women, the triceps and suprailiac sites were the best predictors.

Below are the proper methods of measuring skinfolds with calipers, along with the formulas for calculating body density and fat. Finally, graphs (nomograms) have been included for ease in determining body density and percent fat without doing the calculations.

## Procedures (See Figure 3.4)

1.  First, you need someone to measure you.

2.  Skinfolds are measured on the right side of the body using a skinfold caliper.[2]

3.  Grasp the skinfold between the thumb and forefinger. The skinfold should include two thicknesses of skin and subcutaneous fat, but not muscle.

---

[2]The caliper is designed to exert a pressure on the caliper face of 10 grams per square millimeter. A skinfold caliper that meets these requirements is the Lange Skinfold Caliper (Cambridge Scientific Industries, Inc., Cambridge, Maryland).

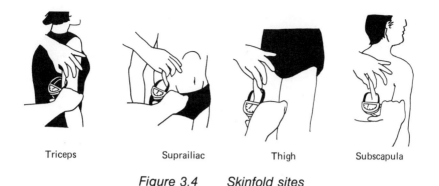

Triceps    Suprailiac    Thigh    Subscapula

*Figure 3.4    Skinfold sites*

4.  Apply the calipers approximately one centimeter below the fingers holding the skinfold, at a depth equal to the thickness of the fold.

5.  Each fold is taken in the vertical plane while the subject is standing, except for the subscapular, which is picked up on a slight slant running laterally in the natural fold of the skin.

6.  The technique of measurement is repeated completely for each site before going on to the next site. This includes regrasping the skinfold. Whenever there is a difference greater than 0.5 millimeter, a third measurement is necessary. *The mean of the two closest readings represents the value for the site being measured.*

7.  The anatomical landmarks for the skinfold sites are as follows:

    *Subscapula.*   The bottom point of the shoulder blade (scapula).

    *Thigh.*   The front side of the thigh midway between the hip and knee joints.

    *Triceps.*   The back of the upper arm midway between the shoulder and elbow joints.

    *Suprailiac.*   Just above the top of the hip bone (crest of the ilium) at the middle of the side of the body.

### Calculations for Body Fat

The formulas below are for calculating the body density and percent of body fat in both men and women. If you are fortunate to have access to skinfold calipers, these measurements will be helpful in providing a good estimate of your relative body fat. Two examples, one for women and one for men, are presented to assist you in your own computation.

WOMEN.

Skinfold Assessment (millimeters)

|  | Trial 1 | Trial 2 | Trial 3 | Mean |
|---|---|---|---|---|
| 1. Tricip | 13.0 | 16.0 | 15.0 | 15.5 |
| 2. Suprailiac | 7.5 | 8.0 | 7.5 | 7.5 |

Computation for Body Density (gm/cc)

Body Density = 1.0764 — (0.00088 x tricep) — (0.00081 x suprailiac)

$\qquad$ = 1.0764 — (0.00088 x _15.5_) — (0.00081 x _7.5_)

$\qquad$ = 1.0764 — (_.01364_) — (_.00608_)

Body Density = _1.057_ gm/cc

Computation for Percentage of Body Fat:

$\qquad$ Percentage Body Fat = (4.570/Body Density — 4.142)100

$\qquad$ = (4.570/ _1.057_ — 4.142)100

$\qquad$ = _.1816_ x 100

$\qquad$ Percentage Body Fat = _18.2_ %

MEN.

Skinfold Assessment (millimeters

|  | Trial 1 | Trial 2 | Trial 3 | Mean |
|---|---|---|---|---|
| 1. Subscapula | 11.5 | 11.0 | 11.0 | 11.0 |
| 2. Thigh | 15.0 | 15.0 | — | 15.0 |

Computation for Body Density (gm/cc):

Body Density = 1.1043 — (0.00131 x subscapula) — (0.001327 x thigh)

$\qquad$ = 1.1043 — (0.00131 x _11.0_) — (0.001327 x _15.0_)

$\qquad$ = 1.1043 — (_.01441_) — (_.01991_)

Body Density = _1.070_ gm/cc

Computation for percentage of body fat:

$\qquad$ Percentage Body Fat = (4.570/Body Density — 4.142)100

$\qquad$ = (4.570/ _1.070_ — 4.142)100

$\qquad$ = (_.1290_)100

$\qquad$ Percentage Body Fat = _12.9_ %

## Nomograms for Predicting Body Fat

Body density and percentage of body fat can be quickly assessed for women and men from the graphs presented below. A straight line joining your skinfold values will intersect the corresponding values for body density and percentage of fat.

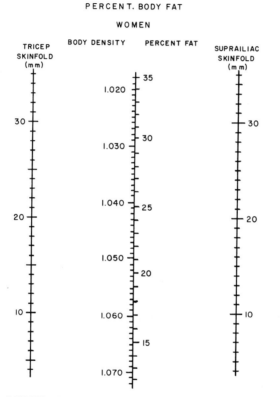

PERCENT. BODY FAT

WOMEN

NOMOGRAM FOR CONVERSION OF SKINFOLDS
TO BODY DENSITY[1] AND PERCENT BODY FAT[2]
1. Sloan, A.W. et al Journal of Applied Physiology 17:967, 1962
2. Brozek, J.F. et al Annals of the New York Academy of Science 101:113, 1963

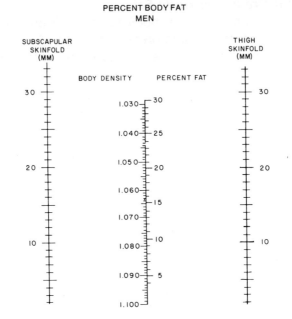

PERCENT BODY FAT
MEN

SUBSCAPULAR
SKINFOLD
(MM)

THIGH
SKINFOLD
(MM)

BODY DENSITY    PERCENT FAT

## Body Fat Norms

A body fat classification chart for college-aged men and women is presented in Table 3.10. Remember, a normal rating refers to the average for the group that was measured. This does not necessarily mean this is the most desired rating.

## TABLE 3.10.   BODY FAT NORMS*

| CLASSIFICATION | WOMAN (%) | MEN (%) |
|---|---|---|
| Very low fat: skinny | 14.0-16.9 | 7.0- 9.9 |
| Low fat: trim | 17.0-19.9 | 10.0-12.9 |
| Average fat: normal | 20.0-23.9 | 13.0-16.9 |
| Above normal fat: plump | 24.0-26.9 | 17.0-19.9 |
| Very high fat: fat | 27.0-29.9 | 20.0-24.9 |
| Obese: over fat | 30.0 and higher | 25.0 and higher |

*Based on the Sloan formulas for young adult women and men.

## Body Build Evaluation

It is natural to be concerned about your body contour or physique and how it compares with others. Regardless of body weight, a body with proper proportions will look better. So what are proper proportions for women? What are proper proportions for men? And how do you rate? Along with knowing your body fat percentage, measuring the girth of certain parts of the body will further indicate the trimness of your body. These figures will enable you to set reasonable goals for yourself.

### *Procedure*

You need someone to measure you and a measuring tape; one made of fiberglass is preferred. The person measuring should apply even pressure on the tape (not too tight) without compressing the underlying tissue. You should stand while the measurements are being made. Take the measurements at the sites described below.

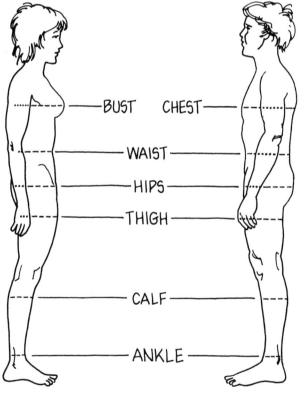

*Body measurement sites*

*Chest.* At the nipple line and at the midpoint of a normal breath.

*Waist.* At the minimal abdominal girth, below the rib cage and just above the top of the hip bone.

*Hips.* At the level of the symphisis pubis in front, at the maximal protusion of the buttocks in back. Be sure your feet are together when measuring this circumference.

*Thigh.* At the crotch level and just below the fold of the buttocks (gluteal fold).

*Calf.* At the maximal circumference.

*Ankle.* At the minimal circumference, usually just above the ankle bones.

*Upper Arm.* At the maximal circumference; with arm extended, palm up.

*Wrist.* At the most minimal circumference; with arm extended, palm up.

The charts below give recommended girth proportions for women and men. These serve only as a general reference based on measurements of many people who we would classify as trim and well proportioned. Record your measurements. After 8 to 10 weeks of physical fitness conditioning (such as jog-walk-jog, conditioning exercises, and maybe modification of your diet), have yourself measured again for changes.

Recommended girth proportions for women:

*Bust* should measure same as hips.

*Waist* should measure 10 inches less than bust or hips.

*Hips* should measure same as bust.

*Thighs* should measure 6 inches less than waist.

*Calves* should measure 6 to 7 inches less than thighs.

*Ankles* should measure 5 to 6 inches less than calves.

*Upper arm* should measure twice the size of the wrist.

Recommended girth proportions for men:

*Chest* should measure same as hips.

*Waist* should measure 5 to 7 inches less than chest or hips.

*Hips* should measure same as chest.

*Thighs* should measure 8 to 10 inches less than waist.

*Calves* should measure 7 to 8 inches less than thighs.

*Ankles* should measure 6 to 7 inches less than calves.

*Upper arm* should measure twice the size of the wrist.

## Determining a Desirable Weight

The following procedures represent a simple way of determining an effective weight for you based on your present <u>fat free weight</u>. For example, let's say a man weighs 200 pounds and his skinfold measures indicate a body fat of 20%. This calculates to 40 pounds of fat weight (20% of 200), or a fat-free weight (lean body weight) of 160 pounds (200 − 40). The latter figure is not his ideal weight, however, because no body can or should be completely free of fat. Referring to the body fat norms, we can take 12% as a desirable body fat level for men. With this figure we can estimate the weight that corresponds to this selected percentage of body fat. In this case, just divide the fat-free weight by 0.88 (100%–12.0% or 1.00–0.12). The result, in this example, computes to just under 182 pounds (82 kg).

This procedure implies that a weight of 182 pounds represents a reasonable goal for the man in our example. For those who have a very high fat percentage, 17.5% or 15% might be a more appropriate first goal. For women we suggest a 18% value as a desirable goal when using the Sloan formula. In this case, the fat-free weight should be divided by 0.82. Below is an example of the computation steps for a 145-pound woman who predicted 28.3% body fat.

Example for Calculating "Desired" Weight.

(1 lb. = 0.45 kilograms)

Computation:

1. Fat Weight = Weight x $\dfrac{\% \text{ Fat}}{100}$

$$= \underline{145} \times \dfrac{\underline{28.3}}{100} = \underline{41.0} \text{ lbs.} \quad (\underline{18.5} \text{ kg.})$$

2. Fat-free Weight = Weight − Fat Weight

$$= \underline{145} - \underline{41} = \underline{104} \text{ lbs.} \quad (\underline{46.8} \text{ kg.})$$

3. Desired Weight at 18% Fat = FFW/0.82

$$= \underline{104} \text{ /0.82}$$

Desired Weight = $\underline{126.8}$ lbs. $(\underline{57.1}$ kg.)

## A FINAL WORD ON MEASUREMENT AND EVALUATION

Measurement and evaluation are very important in our everyday lives. We are always determining the status of the basics in our life. How much do we weigh? How many miles to the gallon of gasoline do we get? Which product is better for our needs? How does the college professor rate as a teacher? In short, we continuously measure and evaluate various facets of our daily living. Through the use of objective physical fitness tests you can evaluate your own physical fitness. The tests suggested in this chapter are all easily administered and have been successful in rating the physical fitness of men and women. The success of the testing program, however, depends on careful and accurate administration of the selected tests. We have tried to indicate the proper testing procedures along with a basic purpose for each test.

As mentioned previously, it is natural to be curious about how you compare with others. We hoped that the results will give you a greater insight into your physical strengths and weaknesses. Consequently, this information can be used to help you develop a plan for an individualized physical fitness program. In the following chapters, training guidelines for developing a *general physical fitness* program, with the major emphasis on cardiorespiratory health, are presented. The need for improving and maintaining a desirable body shape along with adequate strength, muscular endurance, and flexibility is also stressed. Knowledge of your present physical fitness status, as indicated by your test results, will assist you in establishing a beginning point in your program. If you are in doubt about your state of physical fitness, begin your program at the lowest level recommended. You can always adjust upward.

As you progress with your program, you can retest yourself from time to time. How effective has your physical activity program been for maintaining fitness? Where do you stand on the fitness scales? Have you improved? What would be a reasonable goal for you to strive for? These questions can all be answered through a well-organized testing program. Testing should not dominate your exercise program, but it can be a worthwhile motivator to greater effort and to regular, desirable exercise habits.

Examples of physical fitness profile charts are presented on the following pages. In the appendix these same charts can be found where they can be identified by a solid line; they can be removed for classes where the test results are to be handed in to the instructor.

# PHYSICAL FITNESS PROFILE

Date _____

Instructor _____

Name _____ Age _____ Sex _____

      (last)        (first)

Body weight _____ lb   (_____ kg)   Percent body fat _____

Summary of physical fitness evaluation:

| | Raw Score | | T-Scores* | Rating† |
|---|---|---|---|---|
| Muscular strength and endurance | | | | |
|   Grip strength (dominant) | _____ | kg. | _____ | _____ |
|   Sit-ups (bent knees) | _____ | no. | _____ | _____ |
|   Pull-ups | _____ | no. | _____ | _____ |
|   Dips | _____ | no. | _____ | _____ |
| Motor performance | | | | |
|   Agility run | _____ | sec. | _____ | _____ |
|   Vertical jump | _____ | in. | _____ | _____ |
|   Squat thrusts | _____ | no. | _____ | _____ |
| Cardiorespiratory‡ endurance | | | | |
|   1-Mile run | _____ | min. | _____ | _____ |
|   1.5 Mile run | _____ | min. | _____ | _____ |
|   2-Mile run | _____ | min. | _____ | _____ |
|   12-Minute run | _____ | distance | _____ | _____ |
|   Step test (recovery index) | _____ | beats | _____ | _____ |

*T-Scores are derived by converting the raw measurements (i.e. inches, seconds, number, etc.) of each distribution to a common scale of comparable units. Refer to the Appendix for the conversion table, Tables A.1 or A.2. Raw scores to T-Scores.

†To rate each test according to classifiction tables, Tables 3.1 to 3.8.

‡Select only one running test plus the recovery index.

To compute your average T-score for all tests taken, sum the scores and divide by the number of tests completed.

---

(sum of all tests) ÷ (number of tests) = (average T-score)

        A T-score above 55 is considered *good.*

# PHYSICAL FITNESS PROFILE

Date _____

Instructor _____

Name _____  Age _____  Sex _____
     (last)      (first)

Body weight _____ lb    (_____ kg)    Percent body fat _____

|  | Raw Score | T-score |
|---|---|---|
| Muscular strength and endurance | | |
| Sit-ups (bent knee) | _____ no. | _____ |
| Pull-ups | _____ no. | _____ |
| Motor performance | | |
| Agility run | _____ sec | _____ |
| Vertical jump | _____ in. | _____ |
| Cardiorespiratory endurance | | |
| Distance run (perform one) | | |

1-Mile _____; 1.5-Mile _____; 2-Mile _____    _____
(min:sec)     (min:sec)     (min:sec)

To compute your average T-score sum the T-scores for the 5 tests or 3 tests (sit-ups, pull-ups, and distance run) and divide by 5 or 3, respectively.

_____

Sum of 5 tests ÷ 5 = Average T-score

_____

Sum of 3 tests ÷ 3 = Average T-score

Your T-score for the 5 ITEM is _____; Rating _____.

Your T-score for the 3 ITEM is _____; Rating _____.

## KEY WORDS

BODY DENSITY: A term used to describe the compactness of the body and is equal to the body weight divided by the body volume.

CARDIORESPIRATORY ENDURANCE: The capacity of your heart, blood vessels, and lungs to function efficiently during vigorous, sustained activity such as jogging, swimming, and cycling. See AEROBIC CAPACITY.

ERGOMETER: Generally refers to a stationary exercise bicycle that can be adjusted to provide an accurate measurement of the work performed.

FAT-FREE WEIGHT: Your body weight free of fat (often called lean body weight).

FAT WEIGHT: The absolute amount of body fat.

FIELD TESTS: Refers to physical fitness tests performed outside the controlled environment of the laboratory (e.g., 2-mile run and sit-ups).

FLEXIBILITY: The range of movement of a specific joint and its corresponding muscle groups.

LEAN BODY WEIGHT: The body weight minus the percent of body weight that is stored fat.

MEAN: Commonly understood as the arithmetic average (computed by dividing the sum of all scores by the number of scores).

MOTOR SKILL: The ability of muscles to function harmoniously and efficiently, resulting in smooth coordinated muscular movement. A reflection of general athletic skill.

MUSCULAR ENDURANCE: The capacity of a muscle to exert a force repeatedly or to hold a fixed or static contraction over a period of time.

NORM: A standard of achievement as represented by the average achievement of a large group.

OBESITY: An excessive amount of body fat or the state of being too fat.

RECOVERY INDEX: The sum of three 30-second heart-rate recovery counts after the step test.

RELATIVE BODY FAT: The proportion of fat tissue in your body, often expressed as a percentage of body weight. (percent body fat)

SKINFOLD CALIPER: An instrument used to measure selected thickness of fat folds that have been pinched up on the body.

STANDARD DEVIATION: A measure of variability that indicates the scatter and spread of approximately two-thirds of a distribution of scores around a mean (see MEAN and NORM).

STEP TEST: A testing procedure for assessing the heart-rate recovery after stepping on and off a bench for a three-minute time period at a predetermined cadence.

STRENGTH: The capacity of a muscle to exert a force against a resistance.

STROKE VOLUME: The volume of blood ejected from the left ventricle during one heart beat.

T-SCORE: A score that enables you to interpret and compare raw scores from various fitness tests. It provides a simple way to describe the deviation of a test result from the average score for the particular test (see MEAN, STANDARD DEVIATION, and NORM).

## SUPPLEMENTARY READINGS

Balke, Bruno, *A Simple Field Test For The Assessment of Physical Fitness.* U.S. Government Printing Office, 1963.

Clarke, H. Harrison, *Application of Measurement to Health and Physical Education.* Fourth edition, Englewood Cliffs, New Jersey: Prentice Hall, 1967.

Cooper, Kenneth H., "Testing and Developing Cardiovascular Fitness." *Journal of Physical Education.* Special edition: 130-144, March-April, 1972.

Kasch, Fred W. and John L. Boyer, *Adult Fitness Principles and Practices.* Palo Alto: Mayfield, 1968.

Sloan, A. W., "Estimation of Body fat in Young Men." *Journal of Applied Physiology.* **23**:311–315, 1967.

Sloan, A. W., J. J. Burt, and C. S. Blyth, "Estimation of Body Fat in Young Women." *Journal of Applied Physiology.* **17**:967–970, 1962.

Zuti, William P., "Questions and Answers—Testing." *Journal of Physical Education.* Special edition, **164,** March-April 1972.

# chapter 4

This chapter gives the basic principles and guidelines for designing a personalized program for physical fitness. These guidelines are applicable regardless of your age or present physical condition. You will be shown how to regulate your workouts based on your body's response to the exercise workload.

As you read this chapter give thought to the following statements:

• In order to improve in cardiorespiratory and muscular fitness a "vigorous overload" is necessary.

• The exercise heart rate (pulse rate) provides a reasonable indication of the intensity of your workout.

• It takes effort to be physically fit; however, your training program does not have to be at a punishing level to reap physiological benefits.

• Exercise programs at a 75% intensity level, for a minimum of thirty minutes, four days per week, and involving continuous and rhythmic movement will provide significant improvement in the strength and functioning of the heart, lungs, and muscles.

• A workout designed for developing physical fitness consists of three essential parts: (1) a warm-up, (2) a vigorous conditioning bout, and (3) a cool-down.

• After each workout you should feel refreshed and relaxed, rather than discomforted and exhausted.

• Prolonged fatigue for one hour or more after your workout probably means your workout was too demanding.

• Exercise can lead to injuries. Quite often an injury is the result of overdoing it. When beginning a program, it is wise to start out slowly and progress gradually in order to prevent any unnecessary injuries.

# a prescription for fitness

Training and conditioning programs should be tailored to the individual. Nevertheless, the basic principles and guidelines for achieving a desired level of physical fitness are the same for all people. Physical conditioning demands vigorous effort. However, the term vigorous does not mean punishing, exhaustive exercise. In fact, to provide an adequate training stimulus to your heart and circulatory system, you need only to exercise at approximately three-fourths of your capacity for physical effort. Such effort produces a quicker heartbeat, an increased blood flow, deeper breathing, and sweat. Yes, you do need to sweat to gain in fitness, and despite what a recent "best seller" claims, it does take more than 30 minutes a week for the development of total fitness. Such claims are unfounded if you wish to increase muscle tone and improve cardiorespiratory endurance adequately. It is imperative to understand how to begin and how to progress from a light to a more strenuous conditioning workout. Without a clear understanding of conditioning principles, it would be easy to embark on a sporadic and unrealistic program. The result could be unnecessary soreness, frustration, discouragement, and possible danger to your health. This chapter assists you in establishing a personal system for regulating your workouts; one that sets the tempo in terms of what the activity is doing to your cardiorespiratory and muscular systems.

If you are doubtful about your state of health, you should be examined by a medical doctor before attempting a vigorous exercise program. This is very important for persons over 30, and especially important for anyone who has not been physically active on a regular basis.

Furthermore, the fitness guidelines apply equally well to men and women regardless of age or physical condition. Proper application of these basic principles of training will allow you to structure a fitness program to precisely suit your physical needs.

## PRESCRIPTION FACTORS

Much research has been devoted to determining the amount of exercise needed for reasonable gains in physical fitness. Although there is an abundance of information on ways to train, the lack of standardized methods and reporting have made it difficult to recommend any one training procedure. Nevertheless, it is agreed that physical conditioning procedures always involve four factors: *intensity, duration, frequency,* and *type of exer-*

93

*cise.* It is of prime importance to be aware of the role of each of them and its relationship to your present health and physical capabilities.

## Intensity

In order to improve in cardiorespiratory and muscular fitness, a "vigorous overload" is necessary in all conditioning and physical activity programs. During exercise, the heart rate increases linearly with the energy requirement, as indicated by oxygen uptake. For this reason, the exercise heart rate has been used as a simple measure for estimating physiological stress on the body. This measure has been a standard means for determining exercise <u>intensity</u> levels. In 1957, a study of young men yielded a minimum figure for the necessary increase in heart rate. Karvonen, a Finnish researcher, found that to make appreciable gains in cardiorespiratory fitness, the heart rate during exercise must be raised by approximately 60 percent of the difference between the resting and maximal heart rates. Since then, based on more recent research and our own training programs, we have established *an increase in heart rate equal to 75 percent of the difference between resting and maximal rates as a safe and reasonable intensity for most participants.* Basically, calculating a training heart rate is simple. Take the difference between the maximal and resting rates, multiply it by 0.75, and add the result to the resting rate. This is called the 75% *HR max.* Many people can even work efficiently and safely at an intensity of 85% HR max.

An illustration will make this system clear. The maximal heart rate for young men and women generally ranges between 180 and 200 beats per minute. Let us take a maximal heart rate of 180 and a resting rate of 80 as our example. The difference is 100 beats. Seventy-five percent of 100 is 75 beats. Adding this figure to the resting rate of 80, we get a working heart rate of 155 beats; this figure represents 75% HR max, the safe and effective training level for that individual. (see Figure 4-1) Similar calculations for a maximal heart rate of 200 would result in a training heart rate (75% HR max) of 170. Here is a simple formula for arriving at your training heart rate:

THR (75% HR max) = [ (Maximal HR − Rest HR) × 0.75] + Rest HR

The value of vigorous overload (ranging from 60% HR max to 85% HR max) in eliciting a training effect has been well substantiated. Although the complexity of the results makes it difficult to establish a single ideal intensity, from our own experiences in training people we recommend an exer-

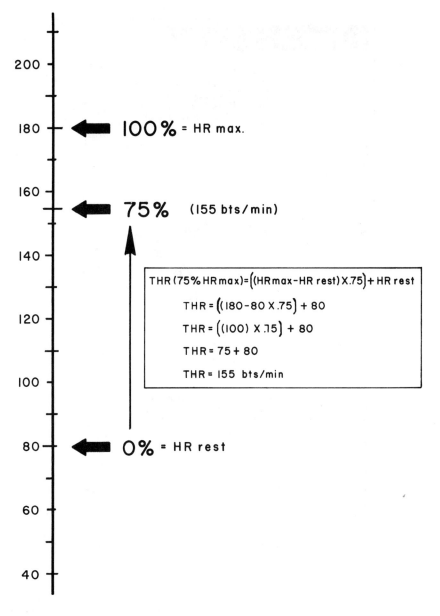

$$\text{THR}(75\% \text{ HRmax})=\big((\text{HRmax}-\text{HR rest})\times.75\big)+\text{HR rest}$$
$$\text{THR}=\big((180-80\times.75\big)+80$$
$$\text{THR}=\big((100)\times.75\big)+80$$
$$\text{THR}=75+80$$
$$\text{THR}=155\ \text{bts/min}$$

*Figure 4.1*

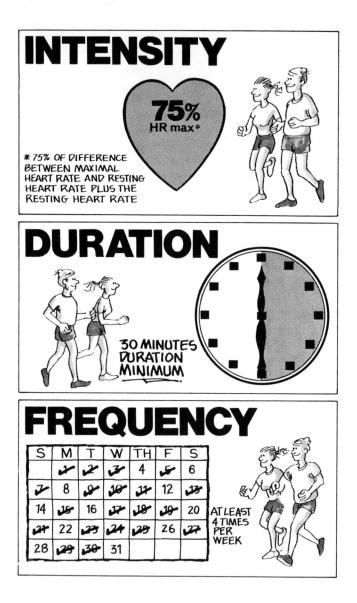

## INTENSITY

**75%**
HR max*

*75% OF DIFFERENCE BETWEEN MAXIMAL HEART RATE AND RESTING HEART RATE PLUS THE RESTING HEART RATE

## DURATION

30 MINUTES DURATION MINIMUM

## FREQUENCY

| S | M | T | W | TH | F | S |
|---|---|---|---|---|---|---|
| | 1 | 2 | 3 | 4 | 5 | 6 |
| 7 | 8 | 9 | 10 | 11 | 12 | 13 |
| 14 | 15 | 16 | 17 | 18 | 19 | 20 |
| 21 | 22 | 23 | 24 | 25 | 26 | 27 |
| 28 | 29 | 30 | 31 | | | |

AT LEAST 4 TIMES PER WEEK

cise level of 75% HR max for producing significant cardiorespiratory benefits. In general, for most young adults, this intensity means a <u>training heart rate</u> in the range of 150 to 170 beats per minute. For older adults, because of a decline in maximal heart rate with aging, a lower heart rate may represent an adequate training stimulus. A rate of 130 to 140 beats per minute may suffice. These intensities indicate safe levels of vigorous exercise for healthy people.

### Determining Pulse Rate

To determine your exercise intensity you must count your pulse rate immediately after exercise. To do this, your first need is a timing device. A stopwatch, a wall clock, or a wristwatch with a secondhand is satisfactory.

Except in rare cases, the number of heartbeats each minute is equal to the number of pulse beats each minute. Therefore, your heart rate can be counted at any convenient pulse point. Generally over the heart, over the carotid artery in the neck, or on the inside of the wrist are the best places for feeling your pulse.

By placing the tips of the fingers on your chest, below and to the side of your left nipple, you can generally pick up your heartbeat after exercise. Your carotid artery (a large artery in your neck) can be located just under

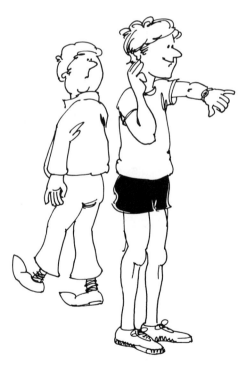

*You need to learn how to count your pulse rate immediately after exercise.*

your jaw bone on your neck slightly behind your Adam's apple. Be sure to press lightly. To take your pulse on the inside of your wrist, place the tips of two fingers, immediately below the base of the thumb. It is important immediately after exercise to find a convenient point for counting your pulse.

When you feel your pulse, count the beats for 10 seconds. Then multiply your 10-second pulse rate by six to determine your pulse in beats per minute. Because of the difficulty of taking your pulse during exercise, for practical purposes it is assumed that the rate counted immediately following exercise is equivalent to the exercising rate. Immediately after exercise, the pulse beats will be faster and stronger and, hence, is easier to locate and count. It will take a little practice, however, before you can consistently obtain a reliable pulse rate.

## Duration

The duration of exercise is directly related to the intensity of the activity. Exertion at a 75% heart-rate increase of the difference between one's resting and maximal rates enables the participant to spread his workout session over a longer period of time than is allowed by more intense levels of exercise. Improvement in cardiovascular function after training sessions of up to an hour or more have been found to produce relatively greater improvements. Existing research and our own experiences in training people suggest that an *exercise session of 30 minutes* is sufficient to produce significant fitness changes.

For a beginning program, however, it is often unwise (and unlikely) for you to continue for 30 minutes at a 75 percent level. At the start, you should limit your workout to a 15- to 20-minute session. You should include brief 30- to 60-second recovery intervals, consisting of brisk walking, between your heavier segments of activity. In these segments of mild exertion the metabolic waste products (such as lactic acid) from your blood stream tend to be eliminated faster than during complete rest. Such intermittent recovery periods also allow you to extend your workout over a longer period of time. Furthermore, they insure that your heart will pump rhythmically at a magnitude well above the resting rate throughout the complete workout.

## Frequency

Regular adherence to a vigorous exercise program is necessary if you are to reach and maintain an adequate level of physical fitness. Thus, don't limit your exercise to physical education classes or weekend recreational activities. Your fitness workouts should be part of your life. Regular, controlled exercise during the week will provide you with abundant energy to make additional weekend recreational activities enjoyable.

Surprisingly, we have found that daily activity, though desirable, is not necessary to improve one's cardiorespiratory fitness. Above-average physical fitness can be attained with *regular workouts three or four times per week.* Keep in mind, however, that improvements in many aspects of physical fitness continue over many months. It is wise to allow several of the initial weeks for adaptation. It must be made clear, also, that this recommendation is based on the assumption that eventually your conditioning workouts will be at a 75% HR max intensity for a period of at least 30 minutes. In our programs, adherence to such a vigorous physical fitness program, for three or four days a week, has yielded physiological and psychological benefits for the participants.

## Type of Activity

Activities that are low in intensity and short in duration produce low levels of improvement. The relative values of various activities for improving physical fitness depend on the physiological intensity required. Golf, bowling, archery, and softball, to name a few, do little to develop or maintain physical fitness. These activities are great fun, but they do not provide the necessary physiological stimulus for developing or maintaining fitness. For similar reasons, Frisbee and backyard badminton cannot be recommended as suitable fitness activities. They simply do not require enough physical effort. However, *vigorous, continuous,* and *rhythmic activities,* such as brisk walking, jogging, running, cycling, swimming, canoeing, cross country skiing and dancing, can be excellent for the development of physical ftness. Why? Because these activities involve movement of the entire body, and they force the heart to beat at a rhythmical rate that is high enough to produce a training effect.

If you have been inactive, you should avoid highly competitive sports, which require sudden bursts of energy and quick movements. The older you grow, the more dangerous these activities become, unless you are participating regularly in a physical fitness program. In general, activities that require short bursts of speed and quick movements do little to improve your cardiorespiratory system.

For example, it is questionable whether 30 minutes of tennis, three or four days a week, will develop a substantial level of physical fitness. Obviously, the skill of the participants will determine the training benefits. Players with reasonable amount of skill will be able to stay active enough to keep their heart rate elevated for conditioning purposes. However, a 30-minute general fitness workout (75% HR max intensity), three to four days a week will produce greater cardiorespiratory fitness. In fact, it can even make one better prepared for the tennis game.

Weight training programs have produced meaningful gains in muscular strength and muscular endurance in both men and women. Although these activities require high levels of energy, they appear to have little effect on cardiorespiratory fitness. The reason is that movement is restricted to specific areas of the body and the activity is intermittent. However, weight training is very beneficial in developing muscle strength and endurance. Chapter 7 shows how weight training can be made part of your conditioning regime.

## VARYING INTENSITY, DURATION, AND FREQUENCY

For some people it may be wise to make slight adjustments of the above suggestions when developing a personalized program of exercise. Age, medical limitations, and/or excess body weight may make it necessary to vary the intensity and duration components. For example, if the intensity is less than the recommended 75% HR max, then the duration of the workout should be increased. Quite often older people or people who are excessively overweight need to start out with walking as the main exercise mode. This results in a lower intensity of exercise, thus requiring a longer duration of activity if fitness gains are to be realized. Research has demonstrated a direct relationship between the degree of cardiorespiratory improvement and the duration of the workout sessions. In addition it appears that a 60% HR max is the minimal threshold of intensity that will provide significant fitness improvement and maintenance.

Likewise, fitness improvement is in direct proportion to the frequency of training. Five-day per week programs result in greater improvements than three-day per week programs. However, since injuries in five-day per week programs are greater, we strongly recommend, especially for beginners, a three- to four-day per week exercise schedule to minimize attrition resulting from injury.

## IT TAKES EFFORT TO BE PHYSICALLY FIT

In our modern world, although nearly everyone preaches the virtues of physical fitness, many of these people do not themselves maintain a regular fitness program. Two primary reasons for this failure of individual fitness maintenance are not knowing how much exercise is enough and the kinds of exercise best for physical fitness. In fact, many writers on physical fitness have neglected to take a firm stand on recommending physical fitness activities. The reader is confused. One frequently hears vague statements, such as, "There are many ways to develop fitness," "Do your own thing," (Choose whatever activity you enjoy. Are golf or archery recommended?), or "Don't overdo it" ("Don't sweat"). These suggestions are chaotic and groundless. Of course, there are different ways to develop fitness. Nevertheless, you must exert yourself (this we call intensity), you must work at a substantial level of exertion for at least 30 minutes (this is duration), and you must adhere to this program regularly (this is frequency). We also know that a total body stimulus through regular vigorous physical activity helps to improve the strength and functioning of the heart, lungs, and muscles. The key to this improvement is the heart rate. It must be pushed high enough and held there long enough for cardiorespiratory conditioning to take place. Let's be clear about it: *it takes effort to be physically fit.* This means giving your body, especially your heart, lungs, and muscles, regular stimulating exercise three to four times a week. This does not mean punishing, exhaustive exercise; it means a workout that is well within your present physical capacity (75% HR max). Not every workout will be filled with joy. The enjoyment comes from a body finding pleasure in its own strength and functional capacity; it comes from a vigor for living.

## DESIGNING A PERSONAL PROGRAM
Very few people have the ability, the capacity, or the desire to achieve the level of physical fitness of an Olympic competitor. Still, many people who wish to improve their own present capacities desire to approach their individual potential, as time and conditions allow. The basic aim of this book is to help you reach and maintain a level of physical fitness that is in step with your everyday living habits. You should strive to live at your physical fitness potential.

Establishing your own meaningful plan requires careful consideration. Your age, sex, and present level of physical fitness will influence your program. Available facilities and convenient activity times must also be considered. Although setting up an initial program is a complex task, the following suggestions will help you design a program based on the intensity and duration guidelines presented earlier in this chapter. Proper application of these principles will enable you to make sensible adjustments for meeting your individual needs.

## The Three-Segment Workout

Most workouts for developing physical fitness consist of three essential parts: (1) a warm-up, (2) a vigorous conditioning bout, and (3) a cool-down. All three segments are essential for a sound program.

### *The Warm-Up*

Proper warm-up before each workout is a wise habit. In addition to preparing your body for the upcoming workout, the warm-up is a precaution against unnecesary injuries and muscle soreness. It stimulates the heart and lungs moderately and progressively, as well as increasing the blood flow and the blood and muscle temperatures gradually. A complete warm-up will stretch the muscles and tendons in preparation for more forceful contractions. It also prepares you mentally for the approaching strenuous workout. You should experience an overall feeling of well being as you complete your preparation. (See page 148 for a suggested warm-up routine)

The time required for warm-up varies with the individual. However, as soon as you begin to sweat (an indication that the temperature of the deep tissues has increased) you are probably ready for the more intense conditioning workout. You should keep in mind that cool weather requires longer warm-up times.

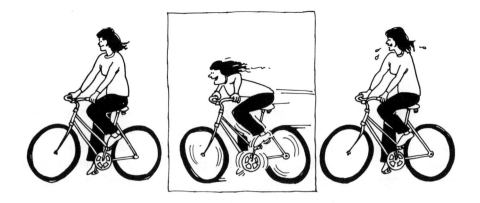

Warm-up          Conditioning bout          Cool-down

## The Conditioning Bout

After sufficient warm-up, you are now ready for the main conditioning segment of your workout. We recommend activities such as jogging-walking-jogging, continuous running, bicycling, swimming, canoeing, cross-country skiing, and other activities that are continuous and rhythmic. However, calisthenics, weight training, interval training, and circuit training are other possible conditioning regimes. On some days, vigorous participation in your favorite sport may be used as your principal workout. (A more detailed discussion of various conditioning methods is presented later in the book.)

In most workouts, your exercise during this vigorous conditioning segment should closely approximate an intensity of 75% HR max as was explained earlier in this chapter (pages 93–98). This figure is sometimes called your *target heart rate*. Note that it represents *your average intensity of exercise.* If you alternate period of vigorous exercise with exercise of lower intensity, you can approximate this average intensity. Your peak efforts should never exceed 90% HR max, however. Generally, rates 10 to 15 percent higher and lower than your target heart rate during your workout will average out to a training heart rate at your prescribed intensity level. On the other hand, if your workout is without alternating periods of exercise and rest, such as continuous jogging or swimming, then your effort should approximate your target heart rate without much fluctuation.

Remember, the key is to tailor your program to your personal needs. As your fitness capacity improves over time, it will be possible to modify your workout and increase the total work accomplished in each session. Always, the duration of the workout should be set so that you feel fully recovered and rested within an hour of its completion. At the start, this duration may be only 20 minutes, but gradually you will become accustomed to 30 or more minutes of vigorous exercise at the intensity level you have established for yourself.

## The Cool-Down

The cool-down is a tapering-off period after completion of the main workout. It is best accomplished by a continuation of activity at a lowered intensity. In other words, keep moving. Walking is the most common means of gradually diminishing your intensity level. Some highly trained individuals use intermittent jogging at a slower tempo as a common cooling-down procedure.

The reason for tapering off is to allow your muscles to assist in pumping the blood from the extremities back to the heart. If you end a workout abruptly, your heart will continue to send extra blood to the muscles for a few minutes. Since the muscles are no longer contracting and helping to propel the blood back to the central circulation blood may pool in the muscles. As a result, there may be insufficient blood for the other organs of the body. In fact, if the brain does not receive enough blood, you may pass out. Thus, it is wise to keep moving to help your breathing and heart rate to return to near normal before you head for a shower. Generally, a five-minute recovery period is sufficient under normal conditions. For most participants, the heart rate at the end of the cool-down should be below 100.

## RELATED CONSIDERATIONS
Up to this point, we have presented basic principles and guidelines for developing and maintaining physical fitness. Here are some additional considerations that will help you in establishing a personal program.

### Activity Selection and Limitations
Activities that don't produce sufficient cardiac stress and profuse sweating are inadequate for gains in physical fitness. For that reason, we can elimi-nate golf, bowling, archery, softball, and other activities of low intensity. On the other hand, jogging, bicycling, cross-country skiing, and swimming are all potentially good activities for attaining cardiorespiratory fitness. Weight training and calisthenics, if properly performed, can do much for muscular endurance, strength, and flexibility. However, these activities are of limited value for developing cardiorespiratory fitness. If played at a high level of skill and intensity, such activities as tennis, badminton, handball, racquet-ball, and basketball can be effective in maintaining physical fitness. But intensity is not the only consideration. Many of these sports require specific facilities such as a court or pool, playing partners and, in some cases, expensive equipment. If you decide to pursue any of these activities, you must consider these limitations if you are to maintain a regular workout schedule.

Let's say your choice is tennis. You first need to find an opponent who plays at your level of skill and who is free at the same time you are. Then you need to find an available court. In fact, if you are a beginner, you should simply forget tennis as a fitness activity. At your level of skill, you will not be able to play hard enough to get any fitness benefits. Play and learn the game, but develop your fitness in another way.

Jogging, along with selected calisthenics for flexibility, strength, and endurance is actually the most adaptable and suitable means for developing substantial physical fitness. Jogging requires no athletic ability, and it can be done almost at any time and any place. It requires little equipment, just gym attire and a good training shoe; most important, it is the most economical activity you can engage in for reaching your cardiorespiratory fitness potential. For these reasons, jogging (along with some walking and selected conditioning and flexibility exercises) is recommended as the basic program for developing and maintaining a good level of physical fitness (see Chapter 6).

Swimming is comparable to jogging for developing your fitness, and cycling, if done for a longer time than jogging and at a high enough intensity level, can provide significant benefits. If you can spare only 30 minutes a day for exercise, either jogging, swimming, or cycling would be a wise choice. These activities can consume as much total energy in 30 minutes as other activities (tennis, badminton, golf) do in two or three hours. This is because jogging, cycling, and swimming will elevate the heart rate to a level that will provide a good stimulus for training and will foster a fitness capacity for enjoying other less vigorous activities to the fullest. In other words, you get in shape to play tennis, rather than getting in shape by playing tennis.

## When and Where to Work Out
Any time of the day or early evening is acceptable for your fitness workout. However, because your digestive system needs blood, it is not wise to exercise less than an hour or so after eating; it is better to work out three to four hours later. Exercise in the rain or cold can be very invigorating, provided you use good judgment. You may enjoy jogging or swimming in the rain, but obviously would get little enjoyment from them during a downpour or a thunderstorm.

Cold-weather workouts are fine, but, frostbite can be a very serious consequence of cold-weather activity. When the air is colder than 20 degrees above zero, the ability to tolerate the coldness is an individual matter. In fact, you may need to find an indoor facility. Granted, jogging is more complicated during the winter than during the warmer months. However, the exhilaration experienced by many people when jogging in the cold and snow enables them to overcome the adversities of cold weather.

Workouts should probably be avoided during the hot and humid midday heat. In the warm months, however, an early-morning workout can be very invigorating. Top off your sunrise workout with a relaxing shower and a balanced breakfast, and you are ready for a productive day. Swimming though, may be your best selection during hot and humid weather.

It is important to choose a definite time of day for your regular workout. Our experiences have demonstrated that a set time for the regular workout will increase your chances of regular adherence to the program. Furthermore, you need a place to work out or to play and practice your sport. Colleges or schools usually have many facilities for exercise. Most institutions have gymnasiums, weight rooms, tracks, athletic fields, and a swimming pool. For people who jog and cycle, the campus and adjoining neighborhoods can also accommodate fitness workouts.

## Clothing

Proper clothing is an important consideration. If swimming is your mode of working out, obviously you need only a bathing suit and an open swimming lane. However, aside from special uniforms and facilities that are appropriate for a particular sport, certain generalities can be made about the proper clothing for exercising and playing sports.

For jogging and other athletic activities, proper shoes are a must. The training shoe (leather or nylon uppers) used by most long-distance runners is recommended for jogging. There are many fine jogging shoes on the market today with good multilayered spongelike soles and a strong heel counter. However, many new companies are now making so-called "running shoes" that sell at bargain prices. Many of these are of poor quality, and everything from blisters to shin splints may be part of the bargain. Although the shoes are supposedly made for running, most of the sales are to people who do everything in them but run. So buy quality shoes from a reputable sporting goods store. Proper footwear is a wise investment. Special shoes are also made for other sports, such as tennis, hiking, and basketball; again, quality purchases are a must.

Your clothing should be light and loose-fitting. Cotton shorts and a T-shirt or blouse are adequate in warm weather. Nylon clothing should be avoided in the heat. Warm-up shirts and pants are all right too; but they should not be worn during hot weather. Avoid the rubberized weight-reduction outfits. These only keep your body heat in and produce sweat; they do not help you to lose body fat. They can be very dangerous in hot and humid weather. Men should wear an athletic supporter or jockey-type shorts; regular undershorts will do for women. An essential part of the female's ensemble is the bra. Sportswear companies have been slow in catering to the active sportswoman. When selecting a bra for activity chose one that has no chafing points such as metal fasteners, hooks, or wires. Preferably the ideal bra has no seams and it should be an all-stretch model pulled on over the head, made of soft cotton, but still providing enough support to restrict bouncing to a comfortable level. Light cotton or wool socks are recommended. Wearing two pairs of socks is not necessary unless you will be making sudden and shifting movements, as in handball or tennis. Eventually you may wish to workout with tennis anklets or even without socks when your feet become accustomed to your shoes.

If you jog or cycle in the winter cold, be sure to wear thermal mittens and stocking cap or wool ski mask. Keep the chest and rib cage warm with several thin layers, one shirt being a turtleneck. For example, wear a T-shirt, a long sleeve turtleneck, another T-shirt, and a nylon windbreaker or sweat shirt. Again, winter jogging and cycling are enjoyed by many people.

## Avoiding Injuries

During the early stages of an exercise program, the chance of injury to the muscles, joints, or ligaments is quite high. It takes time for your muscles

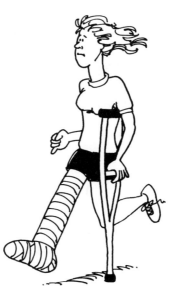

*An injury that limits your workout can be very discouraging.*

and joints to adjust to the stress of exercise. We cannot stress it strong enough. *Do not hurry your fitness program.* Prolonged fatigue for one hour or more after your workout means your program is too demanding. Avoid exhaustion: Your exercise should leave you with a sense of pleasant relaxation and well-being. Generally, it isn't lack of "wind" that slows up beginning training programs; rather it is problems of injured joints and muscles. Thus, your main concern in the early weeks of your fitness workouts should be to avoid unnecessary muscle soreness and injury. An injury that limits or completely terminates your regular workouts can be very discouraging. Here are some guidelines for avoiding injury.

First, warm up properly (See Chapter 5.) Stretch the major muscle groups. Get your heart pumping blood and your lungs breathing air. Avoid sharp turns, and sudden stops and starts, in the early stages of your warm-up.

You should expect some soreness of muscles and joints during the early weeks of your program. These discomforts are a result of the new demands on your muscles. This initial distress should not hinder your daily progress. Eventually this soreness will disappear, to reappear only if you speed up your program, add another exercise, or change sports. Some troubles, however, may be chronic such as knee strain, which is common to cyclists and joggers, and need medical attention.

Avoid jogging or running on your toes. Many beginning joggers try this, but if continued, it may cause soreness in the lower calf muscles. The accepted way to jog is heel-to-toes. That is, first your heel strikes the ground, and then you roll your weight along the bottom of the foot and push off with your toes. In other words, you run almost flat-footed, with your heel touching the ground slightly before your toes. A little concentration on this

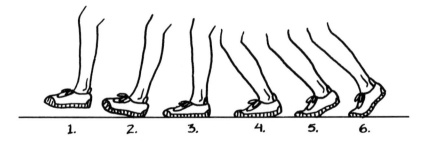
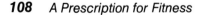

*The accepted way to jog is heel-to-toes*

technique will help you to develop a smooth rhythm and to be mechanically efficient.

Many women have a biomechanical disadvantage when they run due to wide hips, a necessity for childbirth. This causes the leg to swing from a wider distance from the center of running than occurs with a man. This places additional strain on the outside of the leg and foot, and may make the women more susceptible to injury of the hip, knee, leg, and foot. Prevention of injury is the key. When a woman starts a jogging program, she should start slowly as recommended in Chapter 6. The muscles should be built up in order to strengthen the joints of the body. Not only should the key running muscles of the legs be strengthened, they must be stretched regularly. (See Chapter 5 for exercises suited for such development). To repeat, be sure to wear a good running shoe with proper cushion and heel support.

Exercise can lead to various kinds of injuries. Many of these are what we call overuse injuries. Blisters, persistent joint tenderness, inflammation of the tendons and bursas in the feet, and shin splints (low leg pain) are common-occurrences. When these injuries persist, it is wise to seek medical diagnosis and treatment.

**Camaraderie**

We enjoy doing things with others, such as going to the theater, to ball games or on picnics. In fact, much of the fun from these outings comes from our association with friends. So why not plan your workouts with friends who have fitness capacities and activity interests similar to yours. Make it a recreation period of social fun.

For many men and women, exercising with friends has been a key factor in maintaining the fitness habit. Especially, in the early stages of group programs, the presence of others may motivate participants to stay with the program. However, in the end each participant must provide his own impetus and motivation to keep up a regular program. Once you experience the fun, relaxation, and exhilaration that comes with each workout you will not need the willpower or the prodding of others to keep in shape. Instead, you will exercise because you want to and because you enjoy the total body stimulus exercise provides. The company of friends becomes a bonus for your fitness workouts.

**THERE IS NO NEED TO HURRY**

Physical fitness is a lifetime pursuit, so start out slowly and progress gradually. Finish each workout with a refreshed and relaxed feeling, rather than

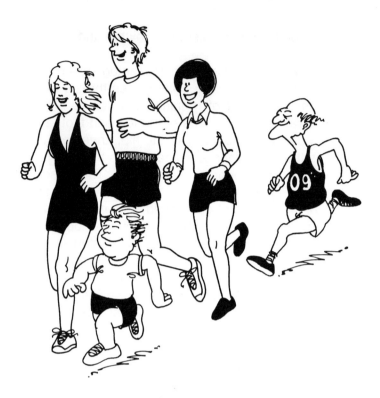

*Camaraderie*

one of discomfort or exhaustion. We have often witnessed a physical fitness aspirant, who, with good intentions, works too hard (runs too fast) and not long enough. Working out at a near-maximal intensity (90% plus) will quickly exhaust you. Therefore, when beginning a program, keep the intensity at a comfortable level. In fact, it is questionable whether hard, exhaustive fitness workouts will produce desirable results any faster than work at a more moderate intensity. A more reasonable intensity allows for desirable physiological adjustments, and involves less chance of injury.

The four chapters of Part II that follow are intended to assist you in developing your own program based on the principles and guidelines presented in this chapter. Basic conditioning exercises and beginning cardiorespiratory programs are discussed in the first two chapters. The next chapter is an introduction to weight training. And Chapter 8 provides suggestions for a more intense type of advanced training for people who wish to achieve an even higher level of conditioning.

## KEY WORDS

CONDITIONING BOUT: The main exercise portion of a workout with a training intensity level at a heart rate approximating 75% of the difference between resting and maximal heart rates.

COOL-DOWN: It is the tapering off period after completion of the main conditioning bout, with activities such as slow jogging, walking, and stretching the major muscle groups.

DURATION: The term used in prescribing exercise that refers to the time length of training sessions. For example, thirty minutes at an intensity of 75% HR max is the recommended duration for developing and maintaining physical fitness.

EXERCISE PRESCRIPTION. Individualizing the exercise workout based on intensity, duration, frequency, and mode of exercise.

FREQUENCY: The term that refers to the number of workouts needed to reach a training effect in conjunction with the intensity and duration factors recommended.

INTENSITY: Refers to the physiological stress on the body during exercise. Your level of intensity can be readily determined by measuring your pulse rate (heart rate) immediately following an exercise bout.

TRAINING HEART RATE: A heart-beat rate (or pulse rate) per minute during exercise that will produce significant cardiorespiratory benefits.

WARM-UP: The exercise portion of your workout that is geared to preparing your body for a more vigorous exercise bout. Generally walking, stretching major muscle groups and exercises that stimulate the heart, lungs, and muscles moderately and progressively are done during warm-up period.

# SUPPLEMENTARY READINGS

American College of Sports Medicine, *Guidelines for Graded Exercise Testing and Exercise Prescription.* Philadelphia: Lea and Febiger, 1979.

Bowerman, William J. and W. E. Harris, *Jogging.* New York: Grosset and Dunlap, 1967.

Cooper, Kenneth, *Aerobics.* New York: Evans, 1969.

Cureton, Thomas K., *Physical Fitness and Dynamic Health.* New York: Dial, 1965.

Pollock, Michael L., "The Quantification of Endurance Training Programs," *Exercise and Sport Science Reviews.* Vol. 1, Jack Wilmore, ed., New York: Academic, 1973.

Subotnick, Steven I., *The Running Foot Doctor.* Mountain View, California: World Publications, 1977.

Wilmore, Jack, "Individual Exercise Prescription." *The American Journal of Cardiology.* **33**:757–759, 1974.

Zuti, William P., "Questions and Answers—Training and Cardiovascular Conditioning." *Journal of Physical Education.* Special Edition: 166, March–April, 1972.

# PART TWO

# DEVELOPING A PROGRAM
# FOR PHYSICAL FITNESS

# chapter five

This chapter provides a selection of exercises for warming up, developing flexibility, and improving general muscle tone. The major muscle groups of your body need to be stretched and relaxed on a regular basis. Millions of people are underexercised. This lack of exercise is a major factor in causing low-back pain and tense muscles. A section in this chapter focuses on exercises for strengthening the low-back muscle groups.

As you read this chapter give thought to the following statements:

• Diet alone cannot keep the body firm and hold the fat in the right places; exercise along with proper diet helps rid the body of excess fat and aids the body in maintaining firm and pleasing contour.

• A sound program of exercise aims at developing all four of the health components of physical fitness: strength, muscular endurance, flexibility, and cardiorespiratory endurance. Thus, conditioning exercises such as the ones presented in this chapter are just one part of a total conditioning program.

• Physical fitness is more than what is reflected in external appearance. In other words, physical fitness represents not only a trim body but a body possessing a good functioning heart, lungs, and muscles.

• The most common cause of back pain is muscle weakness. A program of exercises directed at strengthening, stretching, and relaxing the muscles of the low-back region can do much to prevent or rehabilitate low-back problems.

# individualized conditioning exercises

For many people the word "calisthenics" revives unpleasant memories. It brings back images of tedious, boring, and maybe senseless routines from previous gym classes or athletic practices. The military approach (exercises performed in strict cadence) has never been popular. Nevertheless, a well-rounded physical fitness conditioning program has a need for a segment of calisthenic-type exercise. The exercises presented in this chapter should be done informally at a pace and repetition level that suits each individual. These exercises, if properly performed on a regular basis, will provide adequate stretching of all major muscle groups as well as some strength and muscular endurance development. Despite what many so-called exercise specialists claim, there is no concrete research evidence that exercising a particular spot of the body will take off inches. Inches will slowly come off at the fatty sites when the body's metabolic rate is increased substantially on a regular basis. Doing calisthenics to firm up muscle groups is a reasonable objective but to lose inches of fat with so-called spot reducing exercises is questionable.

It must be emphasized that the selection of exercises to follow do not comprise a total program of fitness. A cardiorespiratory endurance activity is imperative to supplement these basic exercises. Cardiorespiratory exercise (see Chapter 6) such as brisk walking, jogging, cycling, and swimming provide the needed total body involvement that is required to stimulate your heart and circulatory system. In general, calisthenic exercises lack this ability to provide such a stimulus to the heart and lungs.

The suggestions that follow represent a selection of exercises, some of which can be incorporated into the main segment of your fitness program. In fact, exercises for warm-up, flexibility, general muscle tone, and body contour should be part of all fitness and sports programs. These activities provide a means of loosening, stretching, shaping, and strengthening the major muscle groups.

## DEVELOPING A PLEASING BODY CONTOUR OR PHYSIQUE
Everyone is looking for the magic formula to control body weight and to maintain a pleasing body contour or physique. Methods requiring no effort at all are constantly offered to a gullible public who continue to believe there

is a quick and simple solution to these problems. This is the premise on which many health spas or figure salons attract customers. An easily manipulated tape measure assures the "guaranteed loss of inches," rather than the loss of weight. Wrapping treatments for the quick loss of inches or the purchase of equipment that allow you to relax at home as you "tone" your muscles are examples of ridiculous gimmicks that are a waste of time and money. In addition, magazines have always promoted so-called "beauty exercises" for women or the fast, easy way to increased muscle bulk for men.

In 1973 the President's Council on Physical Fitness and Sports published a national survey on adult physical fitness. The major reasons for exercising, according to the survey, were "for good health" and "to lose weight." Especially for women, losing weight and improving body shape are often the prime goals. Diet alone cannot keep the body firm or keep the fat in the right places; exercise is needed to get rid of excess fat and help the body maintain a youthful shape.

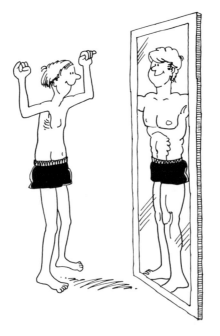

Nevertheless, many men and women believe that physical fitness is reflected only in external appearance. In other words, they have the mistaken notion that if you look fit, you are fit. Few people realize that a trim and firm body, a radiant complexion, and youthful vigor and beauty come not only from exercise that improves muscle tone, but also from activities that stress the circulatory and respiratory systems. We should reiterate that physical fitness, and the concomitant benefits of fat loss and improved body proportions, require a vigorous stimulation of the heart, lungs, and muscles. Conditioning exercise such as calisthenics and flexibility exercises are just one part of a total conditioning program. A sound program of exercise aims not only at shaping the body but at developing all four of the health components of physical fitness: strength, muscular endurance, flexibility, and cardiorespiratory endurance.

**For Women**
The purpose of the basic conditioning exercises is to stretch and firm up your muscles. The best approach for losing weight is to combine these exercises with vigorous activities such as swimming, cycling, or jogging. The myth that vigorous exercise, exercise requiring sweat, is unfeminine, is a thing of the past. There is no adequate substitute for walking, jogging, swimming, and cycling, no matter what the magazines say. Jogging and walking programs that are combined with the basic conditioning exercises result in significant fat losses on the thighs, hips, waist, and arms.

Many women desire to increase their breast size. Because the breasts are composed of glandular and fatty tissue, exercise will not enlarge them. Heredity and weight are the two factors that determine the size of the busts. However, the chest muscles lying under the breast can be exercised. Exercises intended to strengthen these muscles will tone up the chest region and may increase the overall chest girth.

Chapter 3 offers a technique for measuring your fat and girths, and a method for predicting the percentage of fat on your body. In addition, suggestions are made to determine proper body proportions and to estimate your ideal weight.

**For Men**
Whether most men wish to admit it or not, they are concerned about their physique. Lack of chest and upper arm development, too much fat on the thighs or buttocks, or just an overall lack of muscle tone are common

concerns of many men, young and old. The basic coinditioning exercises presented in this chapter are all good for overall muscle tone and conditioning. Weight training is actually the most suitable means for muscle development (Chapter 7). Activities, such as handball, surfing, fencing, karate, and gymnastics will all contribute to total body firmness and development. In short, regular and vigorous participation in exercise and sports will do much for developing and maintaining a masculine physique.

Chapter 3 enables you to estimate your body fat and to determine a suitable body weight. Dimensions for a well-proportioned physique are also suggested.

## BASIC CONDITIONING EXERCISES

On the following pages you will find instructions for exercises that loosen, stretch, and strengthen the major muscle groups of the body. These basic conditioning exercises should be done informally, however, at a tempo that suits you—not as an instructor-led military cadence. The exercises are all designed for exercising the principal segments of the body. The purpose of each exercise is given, and the proper instructions along with illustrations for movement are presented. Also, three levels of exertion (light, moderate, heavy) are suggested for each activity, with the appropriate numbers of repetitions indicated within the circles.

## ARM CIRCLES

| | |
|---|---|
| Purpose: | To loosen and stretch the muscles of the arms and the shoulder region. |
| Starting Position: | Stand with your feet shoulder-width apart and your arms at your sides. |
| Movement: | In each exercise, your arms should make large, sweeping circles. Keep your elbows extended (straight) and swing your arms from the shoulders. |
| *Inward Cross-Body:* | Swing your arms inward, upward, and around crossing in front of the body. |
| | ⑩ ⑮ ⑳ |
| *Outward Cross-Body:* | Swing your arms outward, upward, and around, crossing in front of the body. |
| | ⑩ ⑮ ⑳ |

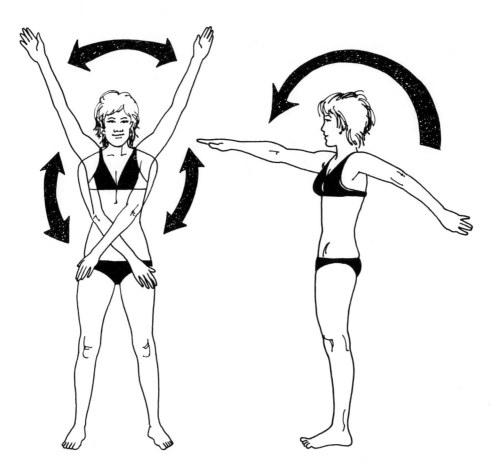

*Arm circles (inward and outward cross-body). Arm circles (forward and backward).*

*Forward:*   Swing your arms forward (as in a crawl swimming motion), making large sweeping circles.

        ⑳    ㉚    ㊵

*Backward:* Swing your arms backward (as in a backward swimming crawl), making large sweeping circles.

        ⑳    ㉚    ㊵

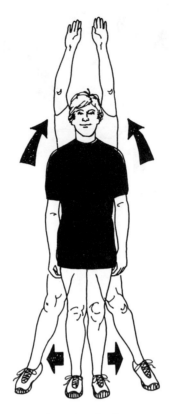

*Jumping jacks*

## JUMPING JACKS

Purpose: To stretch and loosen the main muscle groups of the arms, shoulders, and legs.

Starting Position: Stand with your feet together, hands at your side.

Movement: Jump to a position of feet apart, swinging arms to the side and up over the head. Keep arms straight. Return to starting position. Repeat at a rhythmical and comfortable tempo.

⑩    ⑮    ⑳

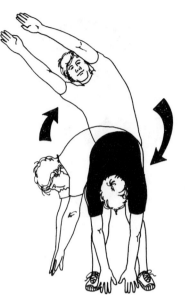

*Trunk bender*

## TRUNK BENDER

| | |
|---|---|
| Purpose: | To stretch the leg muscles and low-back extensor muscles. |
| Starting Position: | Stand with your feet five to six inches apart and parallel to each other. |
| Movement: | Bend forward from the waist, allowing your arms, trunk, and head to hang freely. Reach to touch the floor, then twist the trunk and reach for the outside of one shoe. Hold this position for two second. Return to an upright position by coming up from the side. Again bend forward from the waist and alternate your movement to the other side. Repeat the exercise. Normally, your knees should be held straight; however, a slight bend does not hinder the effectiveness of the exercise as long as you feel a stretch pain in your rear leg muscles. |

④    ⑥    ⑧

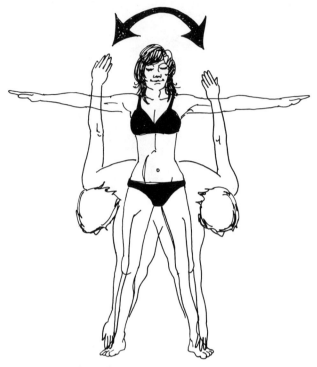

*Opposite toe touch*

## OPPOSITE TOE TOUCH

| | |
|---|---|
| Purpose: | To stretch the hamstring, low-back extensor muscles, and trunk rotator muscles. |
| Starting Position: | Stand with your feet shoulder-width apart, arms extended sideways at shoulder level. |
| Movement: | As you bend forward from the waist twist your trunk and touch your right hand to your left foot, while allowing your left hand to swing high. Return to starting upright position. Then touch your left hand to your right foot in a similar manner. Repeat. |

⑩　⑮　⑳

Your knees should be held straight during this exercise; however a slight bend does not hinder the effectiveness of the exercise as long as you feel a stretch pain in your rear leg muscles.

## TRUNK ROTATOR

| | |
|---|---|
| Purpose: | To loosen and stretch muscles in the back, sides, and shoulder region. |
| Starting Position: | Stand with your feet shoulder-width apart, arms extended to the sides at shoulder level. |
| Movement: | While keeping your heels flat on the floor, twist your trunk to the right slowly as far as you can turn, then return to starting position. Now twist slowly to the left. Repeat the complete movement slowly. |

⑥　　⑨　　⑫

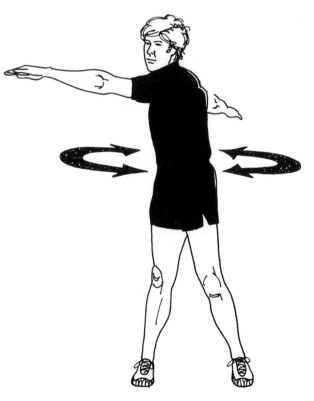

*Trunk rotator*

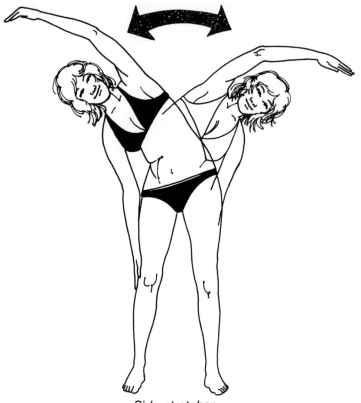

*Side stretcher*

## SIDE STRETCHER

| | |
|---|---|
| Purpose: | To loosen and stretch the lateral muscles of the trunk. |
| Starting Position: | With your feet shoulder-width apart with one arm extended upward (palm facing inward) and the other arm extended downward (palm touching the side of your thigh). |
| Movement: | Bend your trunk to the side of the lower extended arm. Reach with your lower hand and stretch, sliding the hand down your thigh to the knee. The other arm should be stretched over your head and in the direction of body lean. Return to the starting position and repeat the exercise on the other side. Alternate. |

⑥   ⑨   ⑫

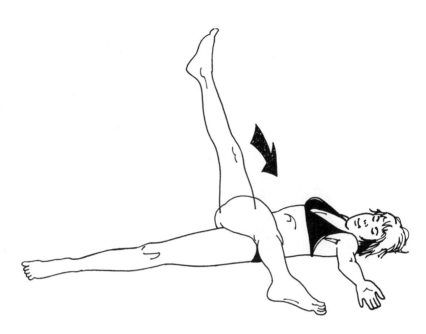

*Legovers*

## LEGOVERS

| | |
|---|---|
| Purpose: | To loosen and stretch the rotator muscles of the lower back and pelvic region. |
| Starting Position: | Lie on your back with your legs extended, and your arms extended at shoulder level (palms up). |
| Movement: | Keep the knee extended as you raise your leg to vertical position (point your toes). The opposite leg should remain on the floor in extended position; keep the back of that leg on the floor. While keeping your shoulders, arms, and back on the floor, reach with the vertically extended leg across your body to the extended opposite hand. Stretch to touch in the area of the extended hand, then return your leg first to the vertical position and then to the floor. Follow the same procedure with the other leg. Repeat the complete exercise. |

④   ⑥   ⑧

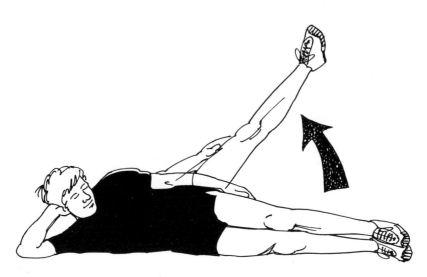

*Side leg raises*

## SIDE LEG RAISES

| | |
|---|---|
| Purpose: | To strengthen and stretch the lateral hip muscles. |
| Starting Position: | Lie on your right side, in extended position, with your head resting on your right forearm and hand. |
| Movement: | Raise your left leg upward from the floor (keeping the knee extended) to a position well above the horizontal, then returning to starting position. After completing your repetitions for one side, repeat the exercise on the other side. |

⑩   ⑮   ⑳

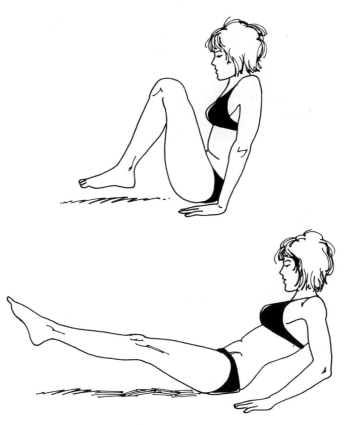

*Sitting tucks*

## SITTING TUCKS

| | |
|---|---|
| Purpose: | To strengthen the flexors of the thighs and the hip region. |
| Starting Position: | Take a sitting position, hands on the floor near your hips, and both knees tucked toward your chest with your heels slightly off the floor. |
| Movement: | Extend your legs straight out from your body with the heels off of the floor, then return to the tuck position. |

⑧   ⑫   ⑯

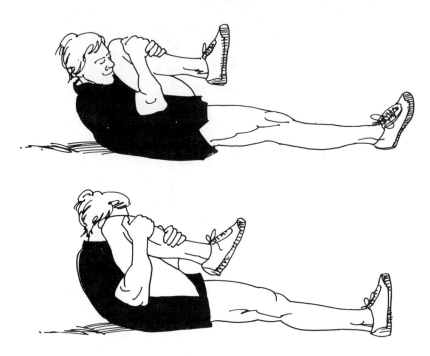

*Low-back stretcher*

## LOW-BACK STRETCHER

| | |
|---|---|
| Purpose: | To stretch and loosen the lower back and hip flexor muscles. |
| Starting Position: | Lie on your back with knees straight. |
| Movement: | Pull one knee to your chest. Grasp the leg just below the knee and pull the knee toward your chest. As you do so, curl your shoulders and head toward the knee. Hold for three to four seconds. Return to starting position and repeat exercise with other leg. Alternate. |

④    ⑥    ⑧

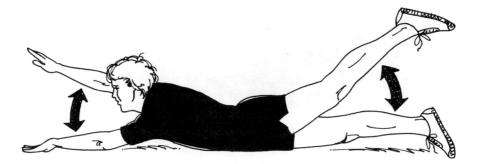

*Arm and leg lifter*

## ARM AND LEG LIFTER

| | |
|---|---|
| Purpose: | To strengthen and stretch the extensor muscles of the back and hip. |
| Starting Position: | Lie face down (prone position) with your arms extended over your head and your legs extended. |
| Movement: | Raise your right arm and left leg simultaneously and keep them extended for a few seconds. Then return to starting position. Now raise the left arm and right leg simultaneously. Alternate. Do this exercise slowly; do not jerk your legs and arms. |

④   ⑥   ⑧

## STRIDE STRETCHER

| | |
|---|---|
| Purpose: | To stretch the lower back muscles, hip flexors, and leg muscles. |
| Starting Position: | Lean forward on your hands, with your right leg flexed under your chest, and your left leg stretched out behind. |

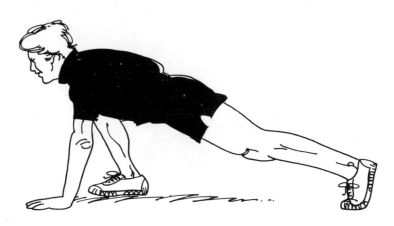

*Stride stretcher*

Movement:     With arms straight and your forward heel on the floor, push your hips down toward floor. Hold for three to five seconds. Repeat the exercise with the other leg forward.

⑤          ⑩          ⑮

## SITTING HAMSTRING STRETCHER

Purpose:            To stretch the hamstring muscles (the large muscles on back of the thigh) and the lower back muscles.

Starting Position:  Sit on the floor, knees extended, your legs spread approximately at a 45 percent angle.

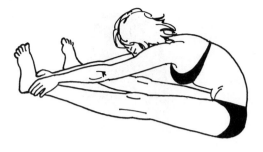

*Sitting hamstring stretcher*

Movement:            Bend forward slowly at the waist. Reach out and grasp
                     an ankle with both hands. Now stretch and try to touch
                     your head to your knee until you feel stretching pain in
                     the back of the leg. Hold this position for two to three
                     seconds, then return to the starting position. Repeat
                     the exercise for the other leg.
                          ③          ⑤          ⑦

## HAMSTRING STRETCHER*

Purpose:             To stretch the large muscles on the back of the thigh
                     (the hamstring muscles).

Starting Position:   Stand and cross one leg in front of the other. The toes
                     of the front leg should touch the floor, heel up.

*This exercise is recommended for the conclusion of the workout during the cool-down period when
conditions are such that you are unable to sit on the ground.

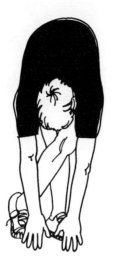

*Hamstring stretcher*

Movement:     Slowly bend forward from the waist, keeping your rear leg straight (heel on floor). Try to stretch until you feel pain in the muscles of your rear leg. Hold the position three to four seconds and return to the starting position. Stretch the other leg in a similar manner. Repeat a few times.

## STANDING HAMSTRING STRETCHER*

Purpose:     To stretch the hamstring muscles and lower back muscles.

*A variation of this is to turn the foot so the toe is pointing to the middle of the body, side resting on support area, and then bending sideways toward the foot.

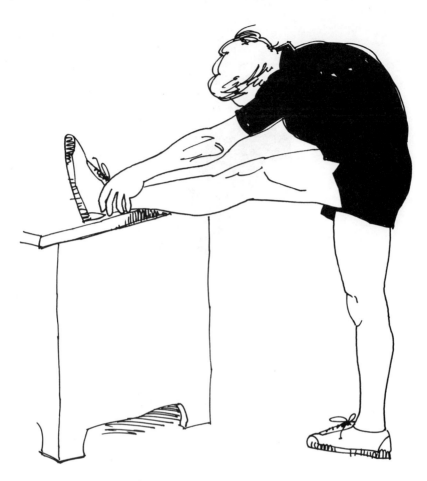

*Standing hamstring stretcher*

Starting Position:    Raise one leg and rest the heel of the foot on a solid object such as a table or chair, toe pointing up. Reach and lean toward the raised foot until you feel an easy stretch and hold for 10 seconds. Be careful not to over-stretch. Repeat a few times and then stretch other leg.

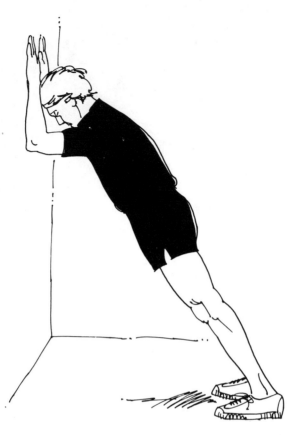

*Achilles stretcher*

## ACHILLES STRETCHER\*

| | |
|---|---|
| Purpose: | To stretch the heel cord on the lower part of the calf muscle (the achilles tendon). |
| Starting Position: | Stand facing a wall an arm's distance away, with your knees straight, toes slightly inward, and your heels flat on the floor. |
| Movement: | With your hands resting on the wall, allow your body to lean forward by bending your elbows slowly. (Keep your legs and body straight and your heels on the floor.) |

\*This exercise is recommended for the conclusion of the workout during the cool-down period.

You will feel stretching pain in the calf and in the lower tendons attached to the heel. Hold for 10 seconds and return to the starting position. Repeat a few times. Do not bend at the hips.

## SOLEUS STRETCHER

Purpose:        To stretch the soleus muscle and the lower part of the achilles tendon.

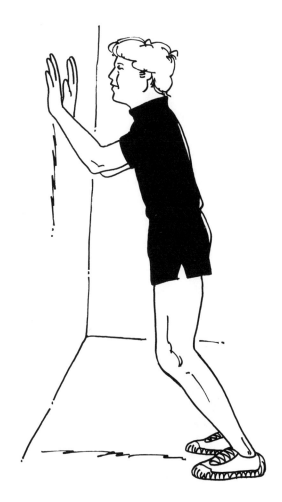

*Soleus stretcher*

| Starting Position: | Stand facing a wall in arm's distance away, bend knees slightly (semicrouch), toes slightly inward, and your heels flat on the floor. |
|---|---|
| Movement: | With your hands resting on the wall, allow your hips to lean forward by bending your elbows slightly. (Keep knees slightly flexed, upper body straight and your heels on the floor.) You will feel stretching pain in the lower calf region. Hold for 10 seconds and rest. Repeat a few times. |

## BACK-OVER

| Purpose: | To stretch the lower back and hamstring muscles. |
|---|---|
| Starting Position: | Lie on your back. |
| Movement: | Bring straight legs over your head so that you are approximately parallel with the floor. Roll back to the position where you feel an easy stretch. Hold this position with legs extended for 10 seconds. Relax by bringing your knees to your ears. Repeat stretch and relax periods for two to three minutes. |
| | A variation of this exercise is to alternate extending and flexing your foot while in the straight-leg back-over position. |

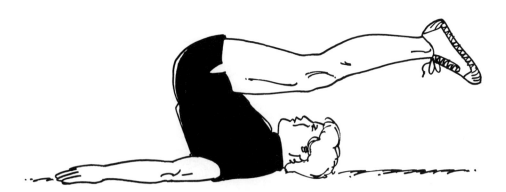

*Back-over*

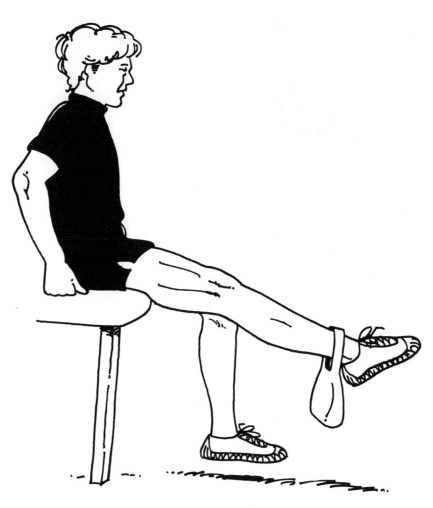

*Quadricep strengthener*

## QUADRICEP STRENGTHENER*

Purpose:         To strengthen the upper front muscles of the thigh (quadriceps), which are the main extensors of the knee.

*This exercise is recommended for joggers and runners to prevent a muscle imbalance due to over development of the hamstring muscles.

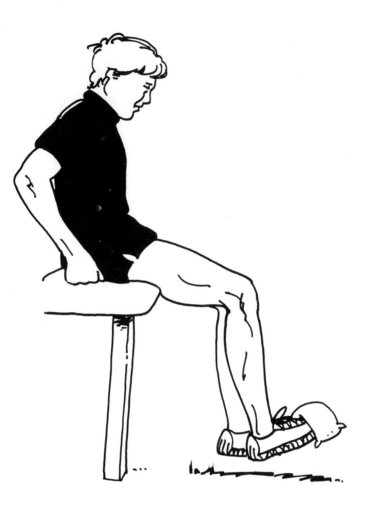

*Lower-leg flexor*

Starting Position:   Sit on a table with legs hanging down. Put a 5- to 10-pound weight over the toes. (A handbag weighed down with canned goods would do.)

Movement:            Holding on to the sides of the table, straighten (extend) the leg at the knee. Hold for 6 to 10 seconds and relax to starting position. Repeat for one to two minutes then do the same for the other leg.

## LOWER LEG FLEXOR*

Purpose: To strengthen the muscles on the front of the lower leg (dorsiflexors).

Starting Position: Sit on a table with legs hanging down. Put a 3- to 5-pound weight over the toes. (A handbag weighted down with canned goods would do.)

Movement: Flex your foot at the ankle by drawing your toes up toward your knee. Hold for 6 to 10 seconds and relax to starting position. Repeat for one to two minutes then do the same for the other leg.

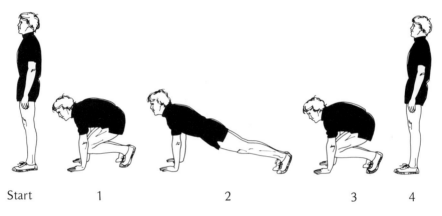

Start      1      2      3    4

## SQUAT THRUSTS

Purpose: An overall conditioner that strengthens the muscle groups of the legs, arms, and body. In addition, it can improve agility and quickness.

Starting Position: Stand with your hand at your side.

Movement: There are four distinct motions to be performed in rapid succession. (1) Bend your knees and place your hands on the floor in front of your feet; (2) thrust your legs back to a full extended position, a front-leaning rest position; (3) return to the squat position; (4) return to erect position. Repeat.

⑥      ⑫      ⑱

*This exercise is recommended for joggers and runners to prevent a muscle imbalance dur to over-development of the rear lower-leg muscles (calves, soleus, achilles).

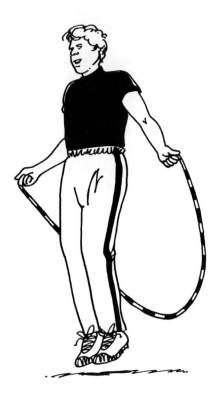

## ROPE SKIPPING*
(See Chapter 6 for suggestions for training with a jump rope.)

Starting Position:    Feet should be close together, weight centered on the balls of the feet, legs relaxed but firm, arms relaxed at sides with rope handles grasped in each hand.

Movement:    Begin by jumping up and down, pushing off the toes, making sure your feet rise no higher than one to one and one-half inches off the ground. As you push off the toes the rope is swirling over the head and comes down under the feet shortly after the push off. Generally, one rope turn for each double jump is a good starting point with 80 rope turns a minute as a reasonable work load. As one becomes more experienced, an

*It is recommended to start out without the use of the rope in order to acquire a relaxed and easy jumping movement.

increase in rope turns and alternating the push off of each foot (jogging step) can be attempted. Many variations of steps can be tried once the basics are learned.

## PUSH-UPS*

Purpose: To develop the strength and endurance of the back of the arm (triceps), chest (pectoral), and shoulder (deltoid) muscles.

Starting Position: Take a front-leaning rest position, supporting your body on your hands and toes.

Movement: Bend at the elbows until your chest touches the floor. Keep your body flat and rigid. Return to the starting position.

⑤ ⑩-⑮ 15 or more

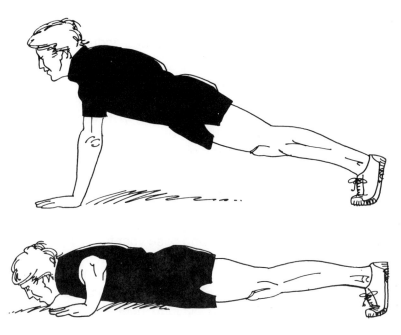

*Push-ups*

*The dip, described on page 55, is another excellent exercise for strengthening the muscles of the arms, shoulders, and wrists.

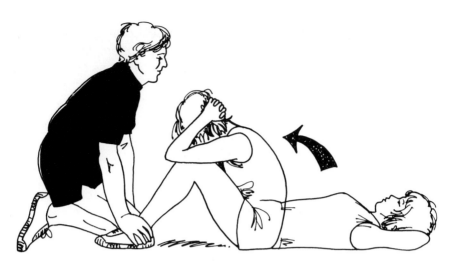

*Bent-knee sit-ups*

## BENT-KNEE SIT-UPS

Purpose: To develop the strength and endurance of the abdominal muscles.

Starting Position: Lie on your back, hands interlocked behind your head. Draw your feet back toward the buttocks until they are flat on the floor (knees bent). The angle of your legs to your thigh should be approximately 90°. A partner should kneel on one knee, placing it between your feet while grasping both of your ankles. If a partner is unavailable, you will need to find a weighted object (such as sofa, mat, or bleacher) to place your feet under for support.

Movement: Curl your back and raise your trunk until your trunk is at least vertical to the floor. Avoid touching your elbows to your knees but, instead, have your elbows go by your knees. Then return to the starting position. Your hands should remain clasped behind your neck throughout the exercise.

(10-16)    (20-26)    (30-50)

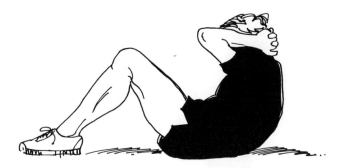

*Half curl-up*

## HALF CURL-UP*

| | |
|---|---|
| Purpose: | To strengthen the abdominal muscles. |
| Starting Position and Movement: | Lie on your back with your hands interlocked behind your head. now bend your knees and draw your feet back toward your buttocks until they are flat on the floor. The legs should be nearly perpendicular to the thighs. Now curl your head, shoulders, and trunk toward your knees, reaching a semivertical position. Hold for 5 to 10 seconds. Return to floor, flatten your lower back to the floor. Relax for 5 seconds and repeat the exercise. |

④          ⑧          ⑫

*If you are unable to do a complete sit-up, you should do this exercise for strengthening your abdominal muscles. Another alternative is to start with your trunk in a vertical position and slowly lower your trunk to the floor.

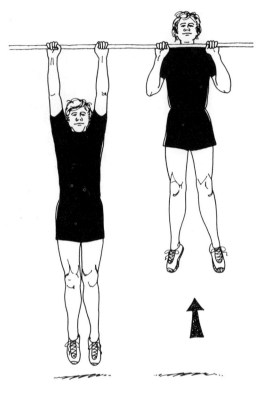

*Pull-up*

## PULL-UP*

| | |
|---|---|
| Purpose: | To develop the strength and endurance of the arm flexors and the muscles of the shoulder and upper back region. |
| Starting Position: | Jump, grasp the overhead bar (your palms facing away), and hang with your arms and legs fully extended. |
| Movement: | Pull up until your chin clears the top of the bar, then lower to a position of *arm fully extended.* Repeat. |

③-④    ⑤-⑥    ⑦-⑧

---

*This exercise requires an overhead bar and, although this has been traditionally a men's test, women can also perform it.

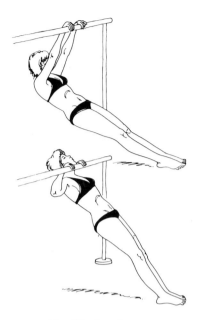

*Modified pull-up*

## MODIFIED PULL-UP*

| | |
|---|---|
| Purpose: | To develop the strength and endurance of the arm flexors and the muscles of the shoulders and upper back region. |
| Starting Position: | The bar should be set approximately at the height of the apex of your sternum (breast bone). Grasp the bar, palms outward. Slide feet under the bar until your body and extended arms form a right angle. Your body should be held in a firm straight position, with the weight on the rear of your feet. A partner should support your ankles during the exercise. |
| Movement: | From the extended body and arm position, pull your chest to the bar. Then return to starting position. Repeat. |

5-10    15-20    25-30

*This exercise requires an adjustable horizontal bar. If you are unable to do a pull-up on an overhead bar, you should do this modified exercise for strengthening your arm flexors and shoulder muscles.

## A SUGGESTED WARM-UP ROUTINE

The following routine is suggested as a basic warm-up for the first part of your workout. The exercises selected have been previously described in this chapter and are designed to exert all the major muscle groups of the body. Emphasis is on stretching the main muscle groups of the body along with some strength and muscular endurance development.

*Walk* (briskly—45 to 60 seconds)

*Jog* (slowly for 35 to 40 seconds)

*Walk* (20 to 30 seconds)

| | | REPETITIONS | |
|---|---|---|---|
| 1. | Arm circles: outward | 10 to 15 | |
| 2. | Arm circles: inward | 10 to 15 | |
| 3. | Arm circles: forward | 20 to 30 | (10 to 15 each arm) |
| 4. | Arm circles: backward | 20 to 30 | (10 to 15 each arm) |
| 5. | Trunk bender | 5 to 7 | (each side) |
| 6. | Trunk rotator | 5 to 7 | (each side) |
| 7. | Side stretcher | 5 to 7 | (each side) |
| 8. | Legovers | 4 to 6 | (each leg) |
| 9. | Side leg raises | 10 to 15 | (each leg) |
| 10. | Sitting tucks | 8 to 10 | |
| 11. | Hamstring stretcher (sitting) | 3 to 5 | |
| 12. | Low-back stretchers | 4 to 6 | (each leg) |
| 13. | Arm and leg lifters | 4 to 6 | (each side) |
| 14. | Push-ups | 5 to 10 | |
| 15. | Bent-knee sit-ups | 10 to 20 | |
| 16. | Achilles stretcher | 3 to 5 | |

Other basic exercises aimed at developing strength and endurance, such as the quadricep strengthener, the lower leg flexor, pull-ups, and more repetitions of sit-ups and push-ups can be added to this routine. Combining these basic exercises with activities for developing cardiorespiratory fitness makes for a solid physical fitness program. (See Chapter 6.) In addition, it is recommended that many of the stretching-type exercises be repeated after the main exercise bout as you cool down and taper off.

## Suggestions for Runners

Jogging and running rate low in flexibility development. In fact, daily running can have some bad effects on the muscles of the legs. Quite often runners experience an abnormal tightening of the back muscles of the thigh (hamstrings). This can lead to strength imbalances, causing injuries. The running muscles, especially the muscles in the back of your legs, need to be stretched before and after each workout. Distance running requires a relatively small range of movement and when the leg muscles are used repeatedly over a sustained period of time, they tend to become very tight. Thus, there is a definite need to stretch the large leg muscles regularly.

The general warm-up routine suggested on page 148 can be used by joggers and runners. However, for people who run and jog regularly, special attention and additional time should be devoted to the hamstring stretchers, achilles and soleus stretchers, and the backover. Such strengtheners as the lower leg flexor, the quadricep strengthener, and sit-ups also need attention to counteract the muscle imbalances that may result from daily running. Again, we must emphasize the importance of stretching to prevent injuries, but most important to counteract the possible bad effects from the overuse of some of the large muscles of the legs.

## ADDITIONAL EXERCISES FOR WOMEN

The exercises previously presented in this chapter are good for improving muscle tone and body shape in women. The following exercises are especially intended for women. They are suggested as additional activities for improving body contour.

## CHEST DEVELOPER

| | |
|---|---|
| Purpose: | To strengthen the anterior chest and shoulder girdle muscles. |
| Starting Position: | Lie on your back, legs extended. Hold a small weight (e.g., a one-pound dumbbell or a small book) in each hand at your sides. Keep your arms extended throughout each exercise. The weights are used to provide a slight load (resistance). |

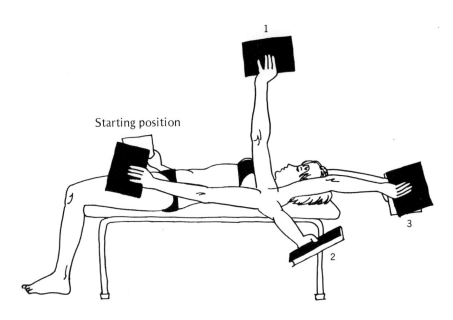

Starting position

*Chest developer*

Movements:

Exercise 1: Keeping arms extended, elevate your arms to a vertical position. Then, lower them slowly to the starting position.

Exercise 2: Bring your arms to the vertical position, then slowly extend them to the horizontal position (arms out to the side at shoulder level). Then back to the vertical position and lower to starting position.

Exercise 3: Bring your arms to the vertical position, then slowly lay them back over the head (extended). Return to the vertical position and then lower to starting position.

*Note.* These exercises may be done in sequence alternating from the vertical position. Also, all these exercises are more effective if you can go below the horizontal, providing for more stretch.

## CHEST AND SHOULDER STRETCHER

Purpose:             To stretch and strengthen muscles of the chest and back in the shoulder region.

Starting Position:   Stand up. Place a light rod (or similar object, such as a rolling pin) behind your back, grasping each end. Now bend forward at the hips, back straight, head up, and feet a comfortable distance apart.

Movement:            Keep your arms parallel to each other and pull them up in back as high as you can. Relax. Repeat the stretch.

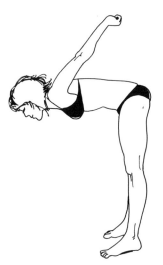

*Chest and shoulder stretcher*

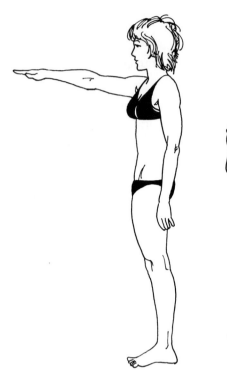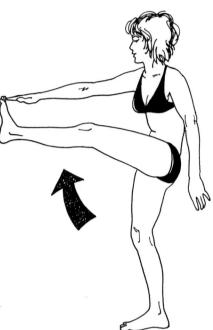

*Kicker*

## KICKER

| | |
|---|---|
| Purpose: | To slim the waistline and tone the legs. |
| Starting Position: | Stand with hands on hips. |
| Movement: | Extend your right arm to shoulder level in front of the body. Kick your left leg with toe pointed and touch the right hand. Your trunk and pelvis will rotate during the movement. After doing four repetitions on one side, repeat the same procedure on the other side. |

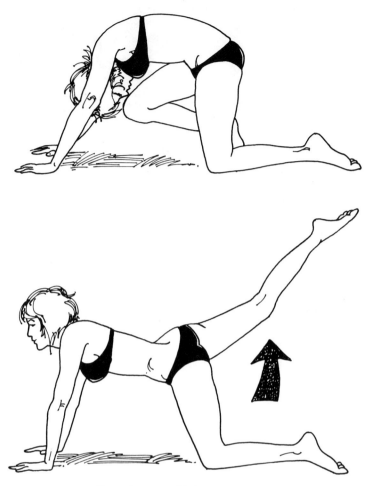

*Knee-to-nose kick*

## KNEE-TO-NOSE KICK

| | |
|---|---|
| Purpose: | To stretch the back, and tighten and round the buttocks. |
| Starting Position: | On hands and knees. |
| Movement: | Drop your head down and bring your right knee as close to your nose as possible. Then, slowly raise your head, and stretch your right leg as far back and as high as you can. Repeat four times, and then do the same exercise with the left leg. |

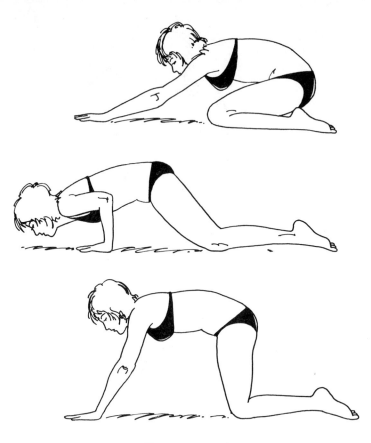

*The cat stretch*

## THE CAT-STRETCH

| | |
|---|---|
| Purpose: | To stretch and strengthen the muscles in the trunk, legs, and arms. |
| Starting Position and Movement: | Kneel with knees apart, your weight back on your heels. Stretch your arms forward on the floor as far as possible. Then thrust your body forward, keeping your chin close to the floor, and bend your elbows. From this position, straighten your elbows and arch your back. Hold your abdominal muscles tight for three seconds. Return to the starting position. |

## LOW-BACK PAIN

### Causes

Low-back pain is a common complaint of many men and women. In general, the back aches because the structures in the spinal region (bone, ligament, and muscle) do not have enough strength to support the weight of the body.

Common remedies for back pain include heat applications, diathermy, or even medication. But such treatments are not directed at the primary cause, which is muscle weakness. Appropriate exercises can eliminate the cause of back pain.

A comprehensive study of 5000 patients, carried out by a combined medical group from New York and Columbia universities, established that about 80 percent of all back pain arises from muscular weakness or inelasticity. Ruptured vertebral disks accounted for less than 5 percent of all cases of back pain.

Since the most common cause of back pain is muscle weakness, especially of the abdominal muscles, exercises directed at strengthening the abdominals and stretching the hip flexors usually help alleviate the pain. Other muscular problems, such as lack of flexibility of the back and hamstring muscles, are also identified with low-back pain.

You can get a meaningful evaluation of the strength and elasticity of the relevant muscle groups in your body by using various tests: bent knee sit-ups and the flexibility tests (trunk extension, trunk flexion) are described in Chapter 3. A poor score on these tests may be the warning signal for future back problems, even if they are not already present.

### Prevention

The lower portion of the spine is a complicated system of bone (vertebrae), muscles, ligaments, and nerves. Not only does the spine have to support the weight of the upper body, but it must be able to bend, stretch, and twist in any direction. Thus it is more vulnerable to strain and fatigue than other areas of the body. When you look at the body from the side, the lower back is normally curved inward, it is not straight. Back trouble occurs when the curve becomes more arched. The causes of this overarching may be poor posture, weak supportive muscles, or even improper lifting habits. Even though millions of people suffer from low-back pain, it can usually be prevented. Good posture habits and exercise routines directed at strengthening and stretching the muscles associated with the fitness of the low-back muscles should be practiced every day to avert low back problems.

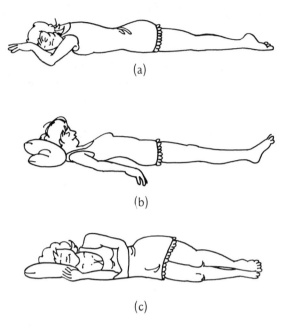

(a)

(b)

(c)

*Figure 5.1*

**POSTURE**   Chronic fatigue and low back muscle strain result from poor posture. The following simple rules of sleeping, sitting, and standing will help you improve your posture.

**Sleeping**   Incorrect sleeping positions can impose a great deal of strain on the back. Sleeping facedown will cause the back to arch (Figure 5.1*a*). Sleeping on your back with legs straight (Figure 5.1*b*) also causes arching. The correct posture for sleeping is on your side, with your hips and knees bent and your head supported by a pillow (Figure 5.1*c*). Another possibility, although not very practical, is lying on your back with your knees flexed.

**Sitting**   A good basic rule for sitting is always to have your knees higher than your hips. When the knees are lower than the hips, the back tends to overarch. When you drive an automobile, you should position the seat so that your knees are above your hips (Figure 5.2*a*).

**Standing**   Standing is very tiring for the back. As fatigue sets in, the hips begin to sag forward. If you are fat in your abdominal region, you will suffer further arching. High-heeled shoes also contribute to the overarching of the lower back. This postural problem can be solved by elevating either foot. Such measures take the arch out of the back. The basic rule is that when you stand in one position for a long time, you should flex one of your hips by supporting one foot higher than the other (Figure 5.2*b*). As long as one hip is flexed, the lower back does not tend to strain forward.

***Lifting*** Improper lifting habits can also lead to serious back problems. There are two key rules for lifting. First, never bend forward without bending your knees. Reaching down to pick up a load with your knees straight

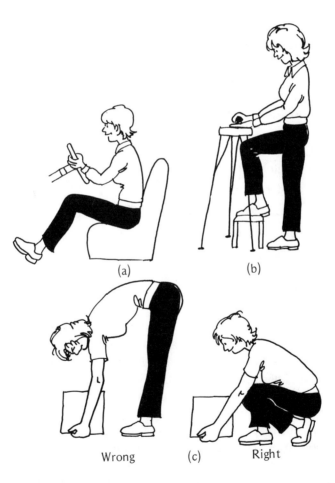

(a)          (b)

Wrong     (c)     Right

Figure 5.2

causes the pelvis to tilt forward and the lower back to arch (Figure 5.2c). Second, never lift anything above the level of the elbows. When you lift an object higher than the waist, the hips rotate forward to maintain balance and the back arches. Depending on the load being lifted, a painful strain can result.

## EXERCISE

Almost all back problems stem from weakness of the supportive muscles of the back; this weakness is the result of lack of exercise. When the muscles are weak, the hips rotate forward, the back arches, the back muscles become shortened, and the weakened abdominals sag and stretch.

Below are exercises for strengthening the back. They were all described earlier in this chapter. It is recommended that they be included in every workout as a sensible means of preventing low back problems.

If you already have low-back pain, you should carry out the following routine two or three times a day. Do the exercises slowly, and as you progress gradually increase the amounts.

### Exercises for the Back

1. Low-Back Stretcher (one knee) (page 130).
2. Bent knee Sit-Ups (page 144).
3. Hamstring Stretchers (pages 132–135).
4. Back-over (page 138).
5. Half Curl-up (page 145).
6. Stride Stretcher (page 132).

### CONCLUDING REMARKS

This chapter was written to aid you in discovering simple exercises that are beneficial for muscle tone and overall body shape. Once you have learned the correct methods for performing the different exercise movements, you can establish a daily routine that suits your personal needs. We should again stress that conditioning exercises, such as the ones presented in this chapter, comprise just one phase of a complete physical fitness program. Despite what many people think, a program devoted exclusively to calisthenic-type exercises will not provide adequate stimulation for the development of cardiorespiratory fitness. Instead, these basic conditioning exercises will help you to warm up, to stretch key muscle groups, and to tone the major muscles of the body. Combining some of the exercises with one of the cardiorespiratory endurance programs we will suggest in Chapter 6 and engaging regularly in one or more favorite sports will provide you with a complete and highly diversified activity program.

## KEY WORDS

ABDOMINALS: The muscles that form the supporting wall for the organs of the abdomen and pelvic regions.

ACHILLES TENDON: The tendon of the calf muscle that inserts on the heel bone.

CALISTHENICS: Exercises and athletic routines for the purpose of muscular development.

EXTENSORS: Muscles that increase the angle at a joint such as the quadriceps extend the knee (straighten it).

FLEXORS: Muscles that decrease the angle at a joint such as the hamstrings flexing the knee (bend it).

HAMSTRING MUSCLES: The large muscles at the back of the thigh that primarily flex the knee.

HIP FLEXORS: The large muscles that are powerful flexors of the hip joint.

LOW-BACK PAIN: The term used to describe the pain resulting from a general overall weakness of the structures in the lower spinal region.

PHYSIQUE: The structure, shape, and appearance of the human body.

QUADRICEPS: The muscles on the front side of the thigh that extend the knee.

## SUPPLEMENTARY READINGS

Anderson, Robert, "The Perfect Pre-run Stretching Routine," *Runner's World,* **13:** 56–61, May 1978.

Barney, Vermon, Cynthia Hirst, and Clayne Jensen, *Conditioning Exercise.* St. Louis: Mosby, 1965.

DeVries, Herbert, "Evaluation fo Static Stretching Procedures for Improvement of Flexibility," *Research Quarterly,* **33:** 222–29, 1962.

Garrison, Linda, Phyllis Leslie, and Deborah Blackmore, *Fitness and Figure Control.* Palo Alto, California: Mayfield, 1974.

Ishmael, William and Howard Shorbe, *Care of the Back.* Second edition, Philadelphia: Lippincott, 1961.

Kraus, Hans, *Backache, Stress and Tension Their Cause, Prevention and Treatment.* New York: Pocket Books, 1977.

Prudden, Bonnie, *Basic Exercise—No. 1.* White Plains, New York: Institute for Physical Fitness, 1955.

Scholz, Alfred E. and Robert E. Johnson, *Body Conditioning for college Men.* Philadelphia: Saunders, 1969.

Sheehan, George, "Six Steps Toward Painless Running," *Runner's World,* **10:** 41, December 1975.

# chapter six

This chapter aims to get down to the specifics of helping you to plan a program for developing and maintaining cardiorespiratory endurance. The paramount emphasis of the suggested programs is to condition the heart, lungs, and blood vessels and to improve the ability to deliver oxygen to the muscle tissue. Continuous and rhythmic activities, that can be sustained over a period 20 to 30 minutes or more, are the best activities for improving the function of the cardiorespiratory system. Jogging and walking are the easiest exercise modes to begin with. However, bicycling, swimming, and other continuous-type exertions can provide an adequate stimulus for developing cardiorespiratory fitness.

As you read this chapter give thought to the following statements:

• The jog-walk-jog technique of conditioning is the simplest method for starting a program for developing physical fitness.

• Minute-for-minute jogging is the most economical conditioner when it comes to getting the most out of the time invested. Furthermore, it does not require extensive facilities, playing partners or opponents, and expensive equipment.

• The key to a personalized program is to establish your own exercise tempo based on your heart rate response to your workout. (Review Chapter 4).

• As a general rule, you must cycle almost twice as fast as you would jog in order to produce the same exercise training heart rate.

• Swimming is an excellent conditioner and even a relatively inept swimmer can get an adequate workout in the water.

• A regulated program of walking geared to gradual increases provides a suitable starting point for people who are overweight, who are older, or who have a history of orthopedic problems of the legs.

• A stationary bike, canoeing, rowing, cross-country skiing, and jump roping are other vigorous activities that can provide a good total body stimulus.

# conditioning for cardiorespiratory endurance

The primary aim of many recent conditioning programs has been to develop and maintain cardiorespiratory endurance. The harmful effects of sedentary existence is reflected in the increasing incidence of premature heart disease. Because our way of life tends to foster coronary heart disease, fatness, high blood pressure, and chronic lung disease, the paramount emphasis in conditioning, therefore, is on the heart, the lungs, and the blood vessels. The evidence to date suggests that prudent exercise habits may prevent these maladies.

By now you have begun to realize the advantages of continuous and rhythmic activities for developing cardiorespiratory physical fitness. Activities that vigorously stimulate the heart and lungs over a period of time and that demand plenty of oxygen will tend to strengthen the pumping ability of the heart and the breathing capacity of the lungs. Because of the ease with which you can establish a safe and reasonable intensity level, we will first recommend a jogging and walking program for beginners. But activities other than jogging can readily be incorporated into your conditioning workouts. Bicycling, swimming, rowing, cross-country skiing, and other continuous-type exertions all can provide an adequate work load for cardiorespiratory fitness. After a good warm-up—a must—you can substitute one of these sports for the suggested routines of jogging and walking. However, you must be reminded that the same intensity level as recommended in Chapter 4 is necessary to produce a training effect, regardless of the activity you choose. Thus the purpose here is to assist you in constructing your own conditioning program for cardiorespiratory fitness.

## A BASIC PROGRAM: JOG-WALK-JOG

Programs aimed at overall cardiorespiratory development use jogging and walking as the main modes of exercise, supplemented by flexibility and conditioning exercises for muscle tone. The jog-walk-jog technique of conditioning represents perhaps the simplest approach for beginning an exercise program to develop cardiorespiratory fitness. The approach presented here is based on more than a decade of successful programs with school children, college students, and older adults. Its fundamental strength is the ease with which individual needs can be met, regardless of age, sex, or level of physical fitness.

There are also many other reasons for the recent popularity of intermittent jogging and walking routines. Specific facilities, such as tennis or handball courts, are not required. Neither are playing partners or opponents; nor is expensive equipment needed. And, most important, you can jog and walk any time that is convenient in your busy schedule. Even bad weather should not hold you back, provided you dress properly and take the necessary precautions. Furthermore, minute for minute, the jogging is the simplest way to begin a physical fitness program. Only 2 hours (four 30-minute sessions) per week are needed for achieving a cardiorespiratory training effect. If you consider that there are 168 hours in a week, this is a small investment of your time.

**Regulating Intensity**

Jogging is defined as a running gait at a pace between 60 to 90 seconds over 220 yards (half the distance around a regulation outdoor quarter-mile track). In other words, jogging is running at a pace equivalent to an 8- to 12-minute mile. At first, jogs of 110 to 220 yards are recommended followed by 55-yard periods of brisk walking. These jogging-walking combinations are repeated throughout the workout. The walking segments are important facets of this continuous rhythmical routine because they represent a semirecovery period.

If a measured track is not available, jogging for specific time segments such as 30 seconds, 60 seconds, or longer followed by periods of brisk walking can accomplish a similar training stimulus.

The key to a truly individualized program is to establish your own work load or, more specifically, your jogging pace. Previously we have recommended the use of your heart rate during exercise as a good index of your overall exercise stress. On this premise regulating your conditioning work load will depend on your heart-rate response. Adjustments in the ensuing workouts, if needed, will be based on your individual needs as determined by the intensity-duration guidelines and principles presented in Chapter 4. The intensity of your workouts should be well within your limits, at approximately a 75% HR max level. Remember the term 75% HR max refers to an increase in the heart rate equal to 75 percent of the difference between your resting and maximal heart rates. Your immediate goal, therefore, would most likely be a heart rate in the neighborhood of 150 to 170 beats per minute. To regulate your exercise intensity, you need to count your

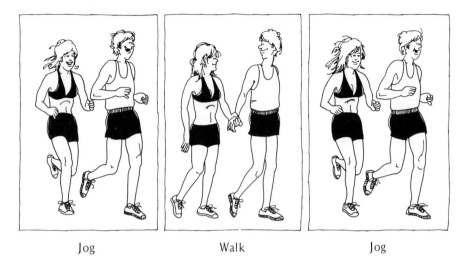

| Jog | Walk | Jog |

*The jog-walk-jog technique of conditioning represents perhaps the simplest approach for beginning an exercise program that develops cardiorespiratory fitness.*

pulse rate immediately at the end of one of your jogs. You will then be able to modify your workout, lessening or increasing the intensity (jogging pace) to suit your needs. Increasing or reducing your jogging time, the distance, or the number of repeats are ways you can regulate your workout. The following recommendations for starting a jog-walk-jog program represent a simple approach to a physical fitness program for all ages.

**The Workout**
A suggested three-segment workout includes a warm-up, the conditioning bout, and a cool-down. The warm-up routine proposed in the previous chapter (page 148) is recommended here. After completing your warm-up, you are ready for the main conditioning segment of your workout, repeated bouts of alternate jogging and walking.

The jogging segment provides the exercise work load that increases your pulse rate to the training intensity level for you. For most people this means a pulse of between 140 to 170 beats a minute. You can either jog for a certain period of time or a predetermined distance. Examples of jog-walk-jog routines are given in Tables 6.1 and 6.2. Each approach is organized in steps so that you can gradually increase your intensity as you improve your conditioning. Note that the distances (Table 6.1) and times

TABLE 6.1.   DISTANCE REPEATS—JOGGING

| STEP | JOG | WALK | LOAD | APPROXIMATE DISTANCE JOGGED |
|------|-----|------|------|------------------------------|
| 1 | Jog 110 yd. | Walk 55 yd. | Start with 8 sets; then in each succeeding workout try to add a set until you can complete 12 sets in succession for 2 days; then go on to the next step. | ½ to ¾ mile |
| 2 | Jog 220 yd. | Walk 55 yd. | Start with 6 sets; then in each succeeding workout try to add a set until you can complete 12 sets in succession for 2 days; then go on to the next step. | ¾ to 1½ miles |
| 3 | Jog 440 yd. | Walk 55 yd. | Start with 6 sets; then in each succeeding workout try to add a set until you can complete 10 sets in succession for 2 days; then go on to the next step. | 1½ to 2½ miles |
| 4 | Jog 880 yd. | Walk 110 yd. | Start with 4 sets; then in each succeeding workout try to add a set until | 2 to 3 miles |

TABLE 6.1. *(continued)*

| STEP | JOG | WALK | LOAD | APPROXIMATE DISTANCE JOGGED |
|------|-----|------|------|------------------------------|
| | | | you can complete 6 sets in succession for 2 days; then go on to the next step. | |
| 5 | Jog 1 mile. | Walk 220 yd. | Start with 2 sets; then in each suceeding workout try to add a set until you can complete 4 sets in succession for 2 days; then go on to the next step. | 2 to 4 miles |
| 6 | Jog 1½ miles. | Walk 2 to 3 min. | After you jog the first 1½ mile and walk, try to jog another 1½ miles or you may wish to jog only 880-yd segments alternated with walking. When you are able to jog a second 1½ miles continuously, go to the next step, continuous jogging. | 3 miles or more |
| 7 | Continuous jogging; Jog 2 to 4 miles. | Cool down: walking. | | 2 to 4 miles |

# TABLE 6.2. TIMED REPEATS—JOGGING

| STEP | JOG | WALK | LOAD | APPROXIMATE DISTANCED JOGGED |
|---|---|---|---|---|
| 1 | Jog 30 sec. | Walk 30 sec. | Start with 8 sets; then in each succeeding workout try to add a set until you can complete 12 sets in succession for 2 days; then go on to the next step. | ½ to ¾ mile |
| 2 | Jog 1 min. | Walk 30 sec. | Start with 6 sets; then in each succeeding workout try to add a set until you can complete 12 sets in succession for 2 days; then go on to the next step. | ¾ to 1½ miles |
| 3 | Jog 2 min. | Walk 30 sec. | Start with 6 sets; then in each succeeding workout try to add a set until you can complete 10 sets in succession for 2 days; then go on to the next step. | 1½ to 2½ miles |
| 4 | Jog 4 min. | Walk 1 min. | Start with 4 sets; then in each succeeding workout | 2 to 3 miles |

TABLE 6.2. (continued)

| STEP | JOG | WALK | LOAD | APPROXIMATE DISTANCED JOGGED |
|---|---|---|---|---|
| | | | try to add a set until you can complete 6 sets in succession for 2 days; then go on to the next step. | |
| 5 | Jog 8 min. | Walk 2 min. | Start with 2 sets; then in each succeeding workout try to add a set until you can complete 4 sets in succession for 2 days; then go on to the next step. | 2 to 4 miles |
| 6 | Jog 12 min. | Walk 2 to 3 min. | After you jog for 12 min and walk for 2 to 3 min, try to jog for another 12 min; you may wish to break this second jog up into 4-min segments alternated with walking. When you can complete two 12-min jogs, go to the next step, continuous jogging. | 3 miles or more |
| 7 | Continuous Jogging: Jog 20 to 30 min. | Cool down: Walking | | 2 to 4 miles |

(Table 6.2) are specified. This does not mean that these times and distances are suitable for everyone. Such factors as heart disease, overweight, and very poor physical condition may limit some people. For those who are overweight (obese) or who are in very poor physical condition, a graduated walking program is recommended as the first step. Such a program is presented later in this chapter. After a favorable response to a walking program, segments of jogging can then be incorporated into the workout program. On the other hand, people who have been more active might begin at a higher level on the listed steps of progression. The load (exercise work load) prescribed for each step in the tables is described in *sets.* One set represents the combination of a jog and the ensuing walk. Graduated repeats of these sets (jog-walk) control and regulate the use of the muscles, joints, bones, and the cardiorespiratory system. If you follow the distance repeats program, a track or running area with a measured distance is needed. However, only an open area suitable for jogging is required for the timed repeats program.

The suggestion to alternate jogging and walking may offend you, because we all tend to see ourselves as capable of greater exertion. And, indeed, you may be! But let's not take any chances. This approach at the beginning will prevent unnecessary injury or soreness, which could terminate the entire fitness program.

After you can handle the suggested work load in step 1 (Table 6.1 or 6.2), increase your exercise work load (e.g., jogging distance) by moving on to step 2. Your aim is to increase the distance or the time of your jogs (maintaining the same speed) until you can cover a mile or more continuously. Being able to jog for two miles or for a continuous time period of 16 to 20 minutes represents a minimal goal for most men and women. Ultimately, your goal is to sustain jogging for 30 minutes per session or for a distance of three to four miles or more. Combining the jog-walk-jog routine with the basic exercises in the warm-up, followed by a proper cool-down at the end will give you a good start on a program for fitness. (See Tables 6.1 and 6.2, pages 166-169.) Remember, jogging is a moderate form of exercise that permits you to work within your own capacity. A good test is to try to talk while you're running. If you can't speak because you're short of breath, then you're probably overexerting.

## BICYCLING

Cycling routines based on physiological training principles can enhance your health and physical fitness. Bicycling outings, whether family get-

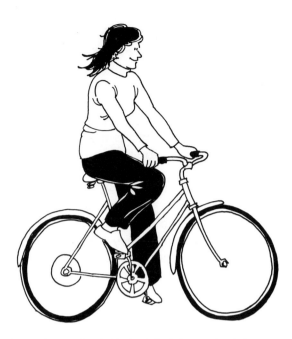

*Cycling routines based on physiological training principles can enhance your health and physical fitness.*

togethers or outing with companions, can be very pleasurable. Much can also be said for the camaraderie and emotional dividends they provide.

Bicycling for physical fitness requires more exertion than is needed in everyday situations like pedaling to the grocery for a loaf of bread. It also requires an awareness of the actions of other users of the road, and a realization of your limitations and the limitations of your equipment. Until you are a practiced cyclist, it is illogical and unsafe to go untrained into heavy traffic, or onto steep and winding roads, or to cycle for long distances.

More than a million people are injured in bicycle accidents each year, and roughly 1000 of them die. Many of these accidents are caused by faulty equipment and poor cycling techniques. The U.S. Consumer Product Safety Commission, in order to reduce the number of bicycle accidents, has set rigid safety standards for all bicycles marketed today. Thus, your first need, of course, is a bike in good working condition that meets the Commission's standards.

After you have selected your bike, adjust your seat to the proper height for you. Many people ride with the seat too low. When you are sitting on the seat, you must have the front part of your foot on the pedal (in the lower position) with the knee joint slightly bent. This alignment places the large extensor muscles in the most advantageous position when you pedal with the ball of the foot.

If you desire to cycle regularly, find a reputable bike shop to assist and advise you. Your bike will need periodic checkups and brake, steering, and gear adjustments. Unless you are quite handy, a qualified mechanic is a must.

Before embarking on a cycling training program, allow yourself adequate practice time to become familiar with the brakes, shifting the different gears, and high-speed riding. The self-confidence you develop in practice will help you to meet actual emergency situations without panic. Many colleges, YMCA's, and adult education programs now offer classes in bicycling that also include mechanical care and repair of your bike. Such courses are highly recommended.

## Training with a Bicycle

To achieve a *training effect* with a bicycle you need to stress yourself adequately. You must cycle almost twice as fast as you would jog in order to produce the same exercise heart rate. Recently, a graduate class project revealed an interesting comparison. Two young men jogging at a 7-minute mile pace had heart rates measured at 150 to 160 beats per minute. When they later cycled over the same outdoor course, they had to ride at more than a 3½-minute mile pace to record approximately the same heart rates. When a young woman jogged at a 12-minute-mile pace, her heart rate was 158. When she rode a bike, she had to ride at a 5-minute mile pace to reach a heart rate of 150, and a 4½-minute pace to record a heart rate of 160. Bicycling can provide an adequate stimulus for training—but this means you must pedal vigorously to stress the heart and lungs sufficiently.

## The Workout

Intermittent activity similar to the jog-walk-jog techniques, either *distance repeats* or *timed repeats,* is a simple approach for conditioning with a bicycle. Distance repeats require cycling a preselected distance (such as a quarter mile, half mile, or perhaps even a mile) at a tempo ranging from a three- to a six-minute mile pace. Your own cycling tempo depends on your fitness and, of course, on your heart-rate response to the cycling work.

TABLE 6.3. BICYCLING REPEATS

| STEP | VIGOROUS CYCLING* | SLOW CYCLING | LOAD | APPROXIMATE DISTANCE OF VIGOROUS CYCLING |
|---|---|---|---|---|
| 1 | 1 mile or 5 min (12mph cycling speed) | ¼ mile or 2 min | Start with 5 sets; then in each succeeding workout add a set until you can do 8 sets. | 5 to 8 miles |
| 2 | 1 mile or 4 min (15mph cycling speed) | ¼ mile or 2 min | Start with 5 sets; then in each succeeding workout add a set until you can do 10 sets. | 5 to 10 miles |
| 3 | 1½ mile or 6 min (15mph cycling speed) | ⅓ mile or 3 min | Start with 4 sets; then in each succeeding workout add a set until you can do 10 sets. | 6 to 15 miles |
| 4 | 2 miles or 8 min (15mph cycling speed) | ⅓ mile or 3 min | Start with 4 sets; then in each succeeding workout add a set until you can do 10 sets. | 10 to 20 miles |
| 5 | 10 to 20 miles or 40 min to 1⅔ hrs of continuous cycling (12 to 15mph cycling speed) | Every 5 miles you may wish to cycle for a mile at a reduced speed. | | 10 to 20 miles |

The cycling speed needs to provide a heart rate stimulus of 75% HR max; the speed suggested may have to be altered to meet your particular training needs.

After each vigorous distance ride, continue cycling at a much slower tempo; this recovery period of slow cycling should last between 30 seconds and a maximum of two minutes. When the recovery period is over, resume the cycling tempo for the preselected distance. (This program is comparable to the jog-walk-jog program.) When you ride short distances (a quarter-mile or a half-mile), your recovery rides should be relatively short (30 to 45 seconds). When you ride longer distances (one mile or two miles) your recovery rides should be lengthened accordingly.

An example of timed repeats would be vigorous cycling for a two-to-four minute period (or, in fact, for any time period in which you can endure and maintain the training heart-rate intensity). Follow this heavy exercise with a recovery period at a reduced pedaling speed. The original exercise is then repeated.

If you gauge your work load properly, either distance repeats or timed repeats will give you sufficient exercise during a 30- to 45-minute session. There are innumberable possible variations in these routines. Obviously it is impractical to present them all here. Table 6.3, however, gives a beginning sequence of workouts with a bicycle for a young adult man or woman.

After you try the workout presented in Table 6.3, you may need to adjust the intensity (cycling speed) to provide a lesser or greater heart-rate stimulus. As you can readily realize from looking at the workout suggestions for cycling, you need at least 40 minutes for an adequate workout on the bicycle. Once you become accustomed to your cycling workouts, you will be able to devise many other workout variations that will be appropriate to your interests and needs. Long distance touring trips (50 to 100 miles a day) are becoming popular pastimes during vacations or on weekends. Whether you tour on a bike or perform a series of timed repeats at 20 mph speeds, you will find the bicycle an excellent device for developing and maintaining physical fitness.

## SWIMMING

Swimming is another excellent means of developing cardiorespiratory fitness. Some people advocate swimming as the ideal conditioner. When compared with jogging, there is less susceptibility to wear and tear on the joints of the knees and ankles. The muscle soreness and tightening, common to joggers, are not usual occurrences among swimmers. The total-body rhythmic movements of all the muscles in a balanced form and the stimulation of the cool water are highly beneficial to blood flow and muscle stimulation. The primary requisites for a good workout are regular access to

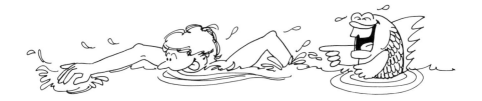

*Even a relatively inept swimmer can carry out a productive workout by swimming.*

a pool and the availability of an open lane; this will enable you to swim unbothered. Even a relatively inept swimmer can carry out a productive conditioning workout by swimming. The only requirement is that one be able to swim at least one lap of the pool.

A simple workout is to swim a length, then climb out and walk back to the other end of the pool, where you started. Repeat this procedure. This is a swim-walk-swim routine similar to the jogging and cycling techniques we have already described. Later on you can increase the intensity of the work load by swimming two lengths in succession before walking a length on the pool deck or resting at the end of the pool. In some situations it may not be possible to get out of the pool to walk. Instead, you will have to rest in the water at the end of the pool. Moderate movement of the legs as you rest will aid your recovery between vigorous swims.

If you are a good swimmer, continuous swimming is recommended. To vary the workout you can swim a different stroke every four lengths. Changing strokes systematically (such as four lengths free-style, four lengths backstroke, and four lengths breaststroke) eases the task of keeping count of the number of lengths completed. Again, if the intensity is vigorous enough, a minimum of 30 minutes in the water per session will provide a physically profitable and refreshing experience.

Table 6.4 provides a sequence of workouts for beginning a swimming fitness program. In this series of swims it is assumed that you will periodically check your pulse rate to assure you are working near the 75% HR max intensity level. Be sure to first warm up with stretching exercises on the pool deck or in the water. Also, you are advised to wear swim goggles to protect the eyes from irritation of the chemicals in the pool water.

Once you are able to achieve step 4, there can be many options: if you have a good swimming skill you can swim continuously for 16 or even 32 lengths (800 yards). However, if continuous swimming is not possible, then

## TABLE 6.4. SWIMMING REPEATS

| STEP | SWIM* | WALK† | LOAD | APPROXIMATE DISTANCE COVERED |
|---|---|---|---|---|
| 1 | Swim 1 length (30 to 40 sec). | Get out of pool and walk back to starting point (30 sec). | Start with 10 sets; then in each succeeding day try to add 2 sets until you reach 20 sets. | 250 yd to 500 yd |
| 2 | Swim 2 lengths (60 to 80 sec). | Get out of pool and walk back to starting point (30 sec). | Start with 8 sets; then in each succeeding day try to add 2 sets until you reach 20 sets. | 400 yd to 800 yd |
| 3 | Swim 3 lengths (90 to 120 sec). | Get out of pool and walk back to starting point (45 sec). | Start with 6 sets; then in each succeeding day try to add 2 sets until you reach 15 sets. | 450 yd to 1200 yd |
| 4 | Swim 4 lengths (120 to 160 sec). | Get out of pool and walk back to starting point (60 sec). | Start with 4 sets; then in each succeeding day try to add 2 sets until you reach 16 sets. | 400 yd to 1600 yd |

*One length is equal to 25 yd.
†In some situations it may not be possible to get out of the pool and walk; thus you may have to rest for 30 seconds in the water at the end of the pool.

intermittent swimming (swim 4, walk and rest 30 to 60 seconds) will be your most logical training method in the water. In general 100 yards of swimming equals about 400 yards of jogging; thus two miles of jogging is equivalent to about one-half mile of swimming.

## WALKING

People who are overweight, who have been very inactive, or who are over 35 may encounter orthopedic problems of the legs when they begin a program of jogging. For this reason, a regulated program of walking geared to gradual increases in distance and vigor is one of the most suitable ways for some people to begin a fitness program. Furthermore, previous ligament or joint problems may be aggravated again if the activity is too strenuous at the start. So, if you are a person who has been very inactive, you

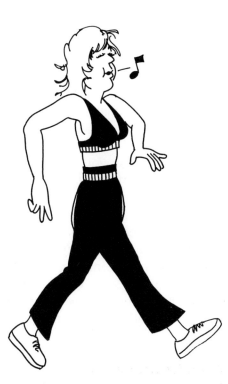

*A regulated program of walking is a suitable way for some people to start a fitness program.*

should consider the following suggestions for your physical fitness program.

To review our basic principle again, your exercise work load must tax you sufficiently if you are going to reap any training benefits. For people with a low level of physical condition, walking can initially provide a very good exercise stimulus. A few years ago we tested an obese student while he walked on the treadmill at a speed of 3.4 mph. His heart-rate response to this work load was abnormally high for this task, over 160 beats per minute. Also, because of his overweight condition, he was expending over 15 calories per minute, which is a relatively high caloric cost for walking. So, for this young man walking was a very strenuous task and it provided a sufficient work load for the start of his training program. The purpose, then, is to provide an exercise stress by brisk walking. The rate of one's adjustment to the walking after a few workouts will determine the readiness to proceed to a jog-walk-jog program. Thus, the following suggestions are for people who are in very poor physical condition because of prior inactivity or an overweight condition.

First, start out walking at your normal easy gait, and keep a steady pace. At first cover a mile if you can. Then, as you become accustomed to the walking try to increase the distance a little each day until you can walk two miles continuously. Check your pulse rate at the end of each walking bout. You may find that your pulse will not be elevated to the recommended 75% HR max level. This is alright because you don't want any ligament or joint problems. Now, as you become more accustomed to the walking, you should increase your walking speed. This may cause a higher exercise heart rate—which is what you want. After you can walk two miles at a good brisk pace, increase your distance to three or four miles. If you find it difficult to maintain a brisk steady pace, periodically slow up for 30 to 60 seconds, and then return to your more intense pace. Eventually you will be able to walk for 45 to 60 minutes at a very brisk tempo. At this point, providing you have no joint injuries or any other health limitations, you should consider engaging in the jog-walk-jog program discussed earlier in this chapter.

## STATIONARY BICYCLE EXERCISERS

For many people a stationary bicycle with adjustable pedal resistance is a convenient means for regular daily exercise. The exercise bike is becoming more common in homes and offices, and some colleges are now providing stationary bikes for their students. For those who are unable to jog because

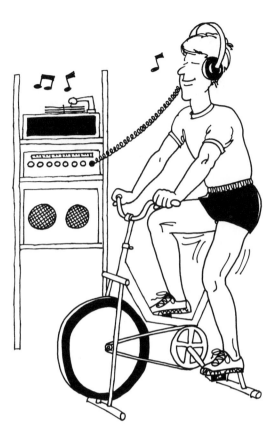

*For many people a stationary bicycle with adjustable pedal resistance is a convient means for regular daily exercise.*

of orthopedic problems, the exercise bike has proved to be a good stimulus for the heart and circulation. One surgeon from our program finds that the exercise bike is an excellent form of relaxation (along with good physiological stimulation) at the end of his busy day. He dislikes jogging, but riding a bike provides him with an opportunity to ponder the day's events and to "unwind" after his working hours. Some people enjoy the stereo or television along with their pedaling routines.

If you understand the principles behind the jog-walk-jog method of training, you can readily see that the same rules apply to training on a stationary bike. Table 6.5 presents a program based on repeated bouts of pedaling followed by short rest periods. Each workout is gradually intensified as you

## TABLE 6.5 TIMED REPEATS—STATIONARY CYCLING

| STEP | PEDALING* | REST† | LOAD | APPROXIMATE TIME |
|---|---|---|---|---|
| 1 | Pedal for 2 min at 75% HR max. | 30 sec | Start with 5 sets; then in each succeeding workout try to add a set until you can do 8 sets; then go on to the next step. | 12 to 20 min |
| 2 | Pedal for 3 min at 75% HR max. | 30 sec | Start with 5 sets; then in each succeeding workout try to add a set until you can do 8 sets; then go on to the next step. | 17 to 28 min |
| 3 | Pedal for 4 min at 75% HR max | 30 to 60 sec | Start with 4 sets; then in each succeeding workout try to add a set until you can do 6 sets; then go on to the next step. | 18 to 28 min |
| 4 | Pedal for 5 min at 75% HR max | 30 to 60 sec | Start with 4 sets; then in each succeeding workout try to add a set until you can do 8 sets; then go on to the next step. | 20 to 32 min |
| 5 | Continuous Pedaling 20 to 40 min. | Walk at the end for your cool-down. | | 20 to 40 min |

*Pedaling at 60 rpm.
†Light walking or moving around can be done here if desired.

adjust to the exercise load. Generally pedal speeds in the range of 60 rpm (revolutions per minute) provide a good pedaling tempo. Depending on the manufacturer, the work load settings are expressed in foot pounds, calories, watts, or on some bikes in kilogram meters. In any case, instructions that come with the bike will assist you in determining a starting point. The key is to set the resistance (work load) at a level that will stress your heart and lungs sufficiently to increase your fitness. Application of the conditioning guidelines presented in Chapter 4 will help you to set up a plan that will provide a very good stimulus for your heart, lungs, and leg muscles. So it is important that you adjust your load to assure a training stimulus at the 75% HR max. (This is an increase from rest of 75 percent of the difference between your resting and maximal heart rate values.) Generally, depending on the type of bike being used, we start people out at a light resistance. If the first workout doesn't elicit a 75% HR max, then we will increase the load accordingly. Always adjust the seat so that it is high enough; the leg in the down position should be almost straight.

## ROPE SKIPPING

Recently, rope skipping has been proposed as a beneficial exercise for developing and maintaining cardiorespiratory endurance. An often-quoted study makes the claim that 10 minutes of rope skipping is equivalent to 30 minutes of jogging. To the individual searching for a convenient and inexpensive form of exercise, this appears to be good news. However, use of basic simple physiological facts questions such a claim. For example, most joggers can average around 10 Calories per minute while jogging (some even go as high as 15–plus Calories).* Over a 30-minute period this calculates to be 300 Calories for the 30-minute session. Now, to jump rope for 10 munutes, utilizing 300 Calories calculates to 30 Calories per minute. This value is above the capabilities of most people. In fact most highly trained endurance runners are not capable of sustaining 30 Calories of energy for even a few minutes.

Our laboratory observations to date indicate that the claims for skipping rope may be somewhat exaggerated. Skipping rope does raise the heart

---

*The value of 5 Calories represents the caloric equivalent for a liter of oxygen used by the body. It is highly uncommon, even for highly trained athletes, to possess a maximal oxygen uptake capacity of over 5 liters of oxygen (25 calories). In addition when one sustains exercise for a period of time, he or she is only capable of exerting at 80 percent of his or her energy capacity. For a highly trained endurance athlete this would calculate to a 4-liter oxygen requirement or 20 Calories per minute. (See Chapter 9 for further discussion on Calorie costs.)

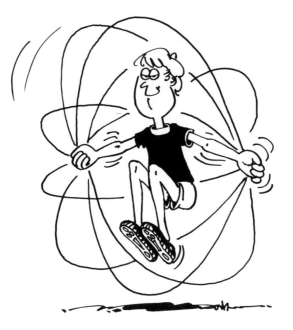

rate substantially, however, the energy expenditure (calories/min), when comparisons are made at the same heart rate, are not as high as the requirements for jogging.

For example, when performed at the same heart-rate intensity, jogging requires more energy than skipping. The reason for this appears to be that more of the total body is involved in jogging than skipping rope. Thus, one is able to do more work at the same heart rate that is beneficial when training the body. Our observations suggest that the metabolic rate (energy cost) for skipping rope is about 8 or 10 times the resting rate. This represents a pretty strenuous activity. Jogging can require anywhere from 8 to 12 times the resting metabolic rate.

If you want to try skipping as a means of training, you need a good rope. It should be long enough to reach from armpit to armpit while passing under both feet. The models with plastic disks that slide around the rope provide a good balance and weight to the rope. Also handles that are reasonably weighted will keep the rope from getting tangled.

If you are out of condition, do not do too much too soon. This, of course, is good advice no matter what form of exercise you choose. Be sure to warm up with some flexibility and stretching exercises. Unlike the jogging and walking programs, jumping rope places a sudden and rigorous demand on the ankle, knee, and hip joints. We have observed that the heart rate for out-of-shape people reaches close to maximal with only one to two minutes of continuous jumping. Quite often they fatigue quickly and have to stop. Even people who are capable of jogging for 30 minutes have difficulty jumping for 10 minutes due to the constant force on the legs. However, it isn't the aerobic requirement (calories used) that tires them, rather it is the acute pain in the leg muscles that limits their effectiveness.

An example of a rope-skipping routine is presented in Table 6.6. The routines are designed to help you progress from a series of bouts to sustaining three 10-minute bouts of skipping. Eighty turns of the rope (two jumps while the rope turns once) is recommended. This rate of skipping will tend to provide a heart-rate elevation close to the recommended training heart rate (75% HR max). For some of you, a lessening of the rate of rope turns may be necessary. As skill is acquired you may need to increase the rate of rope turns to maintain your training heart rate. The key is to progress slowly and avoid undue muscle soreness. You should feel fully recovered an hour after your jumping session. For those who are in reasonable good shape, starting out on step 3 or 4 shown in Table 6.6 may be preferred. In contrast, for those who have been very inactive, repeating a step may be tolerated much better. Remember to progress slowly and avoid unnecessary soreness and injuries.

## CANOEING, ROWING, CROSS-COUNTRY SKIING

Activities involving the arms are known to elevate the heart rate. Canoeing and rowing both require very vigorous use of the arms. To date, there is still argument about the relative merits of these activities for development of the cardiorespiratory system of the average adult. However, competitive rowers have shown to have very high physical working capacities. Thus, it seems logical that regular workouts involving continuous and rhythmic rowing or paddling would strengthen the muscular and circulatory systems of the average person.

Cross-country skiers have been measured at the highest maximal oxygen uptake values ever recorded. This sport requires vigorous movement of both the arms and the legs, and it appears to have a great potential for developing physical fitness in the average person. Continuous touring or intermittent training (similar to the jog-walk-jog routines) on cross-country skis can provide an enjoyable and rewarding workout.

## TABLE 6.6 ROPE SKIPPING (AT 80 ROPE TURNS PER MINUTE)

| STEP | | TOTAL JUMPING TIME |
|---|---|---|
| 1 | Start with 6– 20–second bouts with a 10–second rest interval between each. On each succeeding workout add 2 sets until you can do 12 sets; then go to the next step. | 2 to 4 minutes |
| 2 | Start with 6– 30–second bouts with a 10–second rest interval between each. On each succeeding workout add 2 sets until you can do 12 sets; then go to the next step. | 3 to 6 minutes |
| 3 | Start with 5– 45–second bouts with a 15–second rest interval between each. On each succeeding workout add 1 set until you can do 12 sets; then go to the next step. | 4 to 9 minutes |
| 4 | Start with six 1–minute bouts with a 30–second rest interval between each. On each succeeding workout add 1 set until you can do 12 sets; then go on to the next step. | 6 to 12 minutes |
| 5 | Start with four 2–minute bouts with a 30–second rest interval between each. On each succeeding workout add 1 set until you can do 8 sets; then go to the next step. | 8 to 16 minutes |
| 6 | Start with four 3–minute bouts with a 30–second rest interval between each. On each succeeding workout add 1 set until you can do 8 sets; then go on to the next step. | 12 to 24 minutes |
| 7 | Start with four 4–minute bouts with a 30–second rest interval between each. On each succeeding workout add 1 set until you can do 8 sets; then go on to the next step. | 16 to 32 minutes |

| 8 | Try to sustain skipping for 10 minutes; then rest for 2 or 3 minutes. On each succeeding workout try to skip comfortably for as long as you can, up to 10 minutes. Eventually, your goal is to complete three 10–minute bouts of skipping. | 10 to 30 minutes |

However, the feasibility of cross-country skiing and all of these other activities for your own physical fitness training depends on external factors such as water, boats, snow, or equipment. These needs limit the everyday appropriateness of such activities. Jogging, cycling, swimming and, for some people, walking appear to be the most readily available means for the regular, rhythmic exercise necessary for cardiorespiratory fitness. If you happen to live in an environment that has lakes, streams, or plenty of snow, however, you can derive great pleasure from substituting some of these more specialized activities for the regular ones of jogging, cycling, or swimming. Such activities provide a recreation bonus for the fit, which the unfit cannot enjoy.

## CONCLUDING REMARKS

This chapter has been intended to help you begin a cardiorespiratory fitness program that is geared to your capabilities and needs. We have attempted to provide insight into ways of establishing sound programs of exercises that will adequately stimulate the heart, lungs, and muscles. Programs that can sustain a training heart rate well above the rest rate but not at an exhaustive level have been suggested. These types of total body exercise stress will provide adequate stimulation to the heart and circulation for achieving a training effect. As you progress in your conditioning, you will be able to do more exercise (e.g., jog farther) at the same training heart rate, an indication that you are improving. Remember, these suggestions are not ironclad; rather, they are examples of workable programs that can be easily modified to suit your individual needs. Adherence to these programs have benefited people in the past, and we see no reason why you cannot be successful with them.

After you begin to notice some improvement, you may wish to retest yourself on some of the cardiorespiratory fitness tests suggested in Chapter 3. For example, if you are a woman, the time it takes you to run one and

one-half miles can give you some indication of your improvement in cardiorespiratory fitness. The two-mile run will also provide a good estimation
for men (refer to the classification charts on pages 68, 69, 72 and 73).

The development of strength and muscular endurance with weight training is the topic for the next chapter. This is followed in Chapter 8 by more
advanced training methods for cardiorespiratory development (interval
and continuous training) and an individualized all-around program, circuit
training.

## KEY WORDS

CARDIORESPIRATORY FITNESS: The efficient functioning and health of
the circulatory and respiratory systems.

DISTANCE REPEATS: The repeated bouts of alternate jogging and walking using specified distances as the determinant of the work load.

EXERCISE PRESCRIPTION: Individualizing the exercise workout based
on intensity, duration, frequency, and mode of exercise.

INTENSITY: The physiological stress on the body during exercise. Your
level of intensity can be determined by measuring your pulse rate
(heart rate) immediately following an exercise bout.

TIMED REPEATS: The repeated bouts of alternate jogging and walking
using time as the determinant of the work load.

TRAINING EFFECT: The term used to describe the many physiological
changes that result from participation in vigorous, muscular fitness
activities.

TRAINING HEART RATE: A heart beat rate (or pulse rate) per minute
during exercise that will produce significant cardiorespiratory benefits.

## SUPPLEMENTARY READINGS

*Aqua Dynamics,* President's Council of Physical Fitness and Sports.
Washington, D.C.: U.S. Government Printing Office, 1977.

Bowerman, William J. and W. E. Harris, *Jogging.* New York: Grosset & Dunlap, 1967.

Fixx, James F., *The Complete Book of Running.* New York: Random House, 1977.

Roby, Frederick B. and Russell P. Davis, *Jogging for Fitness and Weight Control.* Philadelphia: Saunders, 1970.

Runner's World Magazine, *The Female Runner.* Mountain View, California: World Publications, 1974.

Ryan, Allan J. (Moderator), "How Good is Bike Riding as Primary Exercise," *The Physician and Sportsmedicine,* **3:** 37, April 1975.

Shepro, David and Howard G. Knuttgen, *Complete Conditioning: The No-nonsense Guide to Fitness and Good health.* Phillippines: Addison-Wesley, 1976.

Ullyot, Joan, *Women's Running.* Mountain View California: World Publications, 1977.

# chapter seven

A muscle must be overloaded to be strengthened. Weight training is a basic and effective means for developing strength and muscular endurance. Everday living does not require regular stimulation to the muscle tissue for adequately overloading the major muscle groups of the body. Thus, weight training represents a reasonable approach for men and women to improve both muscular strength and endurance.

As you read this chapter give thought to the following statements:

• Isotonic type exercises (movement) have several advantages over isometric exercises (no movement).

• Strength improvements are gained when the muscle is stressed systematically and progressively to a greater-than-normal load.

• The degree of strength improvement is directly related to the degree of overload.

• Women who work out on a regular basis with weight training tend not to reflect the increase in muscle bulk observed so often in men who train with weights.

• Generally, three training sessions a week with weights and barbells will lead to significant strength gains in six to eight weeks.

• Weight training programs when not supplemented with cardiorespiratory training are not adequate for developing and maintaining a quality fitness level of the heart, lungs, and blood vessels.

• Isokinetics represent a new concept of strength development by which you either push or pull against a mechanism, and it resists with the exact force that you apply. Simply put, the amount of resistance created by the isokinetic apparatus always equals the amount of force being applied by the muscle.

# weight training

Strength, power, and muscular endurance are valuable assets in many everyday activities, and they provide a foundation for successful participation in sports. Strength is the capacity of a muscle to exert a maximal force against a resistance. It is related to power, which is the rate at which force can be produced. In most athletic activities, power, the explosive ability to apply force is paramount. Muscular endurance is the capacity of a muscle to exert a force repeatedly over a period of time, or to apply strength and sustain it. It is important not only to be able to apply force (strength), or to apply force with speed (power), but also be able to sustain this force over a period of time (endurance).

Weight training is an effective means of developing strength and muscular endurance. A muscle must be overloaded to be strengthened. If not, it weakens. Since our everyday activity does not require such an overload, we need to provide regular muscle stimulation for body strength and endurance. The suggested weight training program that follows is intended for both men and women. Basic exercises are given for all the major muscle groups with the aim of improving both general muscular strength and endurance.

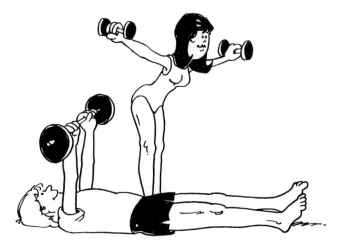

*Weight training is an effective means of developing strength and muscular endurance.*

**189**

## IMPROVING STRENGTH

Much research has been devoted to finding methods for improving muscular strength and endurance. These traits can be readily improved in most people, but there is disagreement over the relative merits of two different kinds of programs, isotonic and isometric. An isotonic (dynamic) contraction is the normal way a muscle shortens when lifting a load. In an isometric (static) contraction, by contrast, the muscle contracts but its overall length is not permitted to change. This kind of contraction occurs when we press or pull against an immovable object.

Recently isokinetics, a third type of strength-developing program has emerged. This program makes use of specialized apparatus to provide a maximal resistance to the muscles throughout a full range of their movement. However, because of the need for this equipment, isokinetic exercise is not feasible for the average person. Nevertheless, in the last section of this chapter, we explain this *new* approach to strength training in greater detail.

All things considered, the use of barbells still remains the most economical means for enhancing muscle tone, strength, and endurance. However, it is speculated that as isokinetic equipment becomes more readily available to the masses, isokinetic training will be the program of the future for developing strength.

### Isotonic Versus Isometric

Until fairly recently, programs for increasing strength were usually based on some form of isotonic contraction, such as lifting barbells. In 1953, however, German researchers published a report indicating that significant gains in strength could be obtained from isometric training. These findings gave rise to a dispute over the merits of the two contrasting methods. After many further studies in which direct comparisons were made, isotonic progressive resistance programs (such as weight training) emerged as the most favorable means for developing muscular strength and endurance. Both methods can produce significant gains in strength in short periods of time. However, isotonic exercises involve the full range of the muscle's motion in one contraction, whereas several isometric contractions are required, at different angles, to produce the same result. Isotonic exercises, when performed through the complete range of motion, can also enhance flexibility. In addition, they develop a greater muscular endurance than isometrics do. Furthermore, the dynamic movement of isotonic exercises may offer a psychological advantage: one is able to see the work being accomplished instead of straining against an immovable object.

In view of the several advantages of isotonic over isometric exercise, we do not hesitate to recommend isotonic weight training routines as a sound means for developing strength and muscular endurance in both men and women.

### The Overload Principle

The development of strength results from an increase in the thickness of the muscle fibers within a muscle rather than from an increase in their number. The increase in fiber size is termed hypertrophy. Hypertrophy and the corresponding improvements in strength are produced by subjecting the muscle to a greater-than-normal load. This is known as the overload principle.

Systematic and progressive overloading of a muscle increases its strength. Generally, the degree of improvement is directly related to the degree of overload. Once a muscle has adapted to a higher demand, an additional increase in the load is necessary to produce further gains. In progressive-resistance exercises (such as training with barbells and weights) the muscle is called on to contract against a resistance that requires a maximal or near-maximal contraction.

The beneficial effects of progressive-resistance exercise programs have been demonstrated in both men and, more recently, women. Many women fear that exercise with barbells and weights will make them heavily muscled and unfeminine-looking. There is no scientific basis to this fear. Women normally have less muscle mass than men. However, there is as much variance among women in muscle-mass development as there is among men. Thus, it is quite possible for some women to be stronger than some men. The inherent capacity for muscle development, however, is genetically determined by the sex hormone levels. The male hormone, testosterone, is responsible for muscle bulkiness in males. This hormone is present in women, but in amounts that are probably too low to have a substantial effect on muscle size.

Dr. Jack Wilmore, an exercise physiologist, has studied this phenomenon. He compared the increases in strength of college-aged men and women after a 10-week weight training program. The women made substantial gains in strength, as did the men. When leg strength was expressed relative to body weight (leg strength/body weight), the values for women and men were almost identical. However, the women's muscle size increased little more than half as much as the men's. Wilmore's findings support the theory that women can increase their strength significantly without—and this is perhaps most important to the female exerciser—a corresponding increase in muscle bulk. Thus, weight training in women seems to produce not bulky, masculine muscles, but rather a trim, well-contoured figure. Dr. Wilmore also concludes from his research that women's strength potential is proportional to men's, once differences in body size are taken into account. Thus a woman can both improve her strength and enhance her figure through weight-training activities.

## A WEIGHT TRAINING PROGRAM
A basic weight training program should systematically involve all the major muscle groups of the body. The proper use of weights will increase not only strength and endurance, but also flexibility and power. Although weight training is a vigorous activity, this form of exercise does not significantly improve cardiorespiratory endurance. However, it does provide an important supplement to cardiorespiratory fitness activities such as jogging, cycling, or swimming.

### Basic Equipment
The beginning program that we present in this chapter requires the use of a barbell and weighted plates. This equipment can be purchased at most sporting goods stores. The barbell is a steel bar five to six feet long with a collar for holding the weights in place at each end of the bar. Standard sets usually contain 2½-, 5-, 10-, and 25-pound weighted plates for each end. Normally the barbell and collars together weigh around 25 pounds. The number of weighted plates required depends on the type of program. The average young adult male needs about 175 pounds of weights for the bar. For women, 100 pounds appears to be sufficient.

A sturdy bench is needed if the bench press is to be included in the exercise routine. Additional equipment such as dumbbells, pulley weights, weighted shoes, to name a few, can add variety to a program. The bibliography at the end of this chapter suggests some comprehensive writings that provide detailed information on the use of such accessory equipment.

### Weight Training Terminology
Some basic terminology is necessary for understanding the procedures and techniques of weight training. The term <u>repetitions</u> refers to the number

of contractions per bout, or set. For instance, if you curl a barbell six consecutive times, you have completed one set of six repetitions (reps). The total poundage (bar, plates, and collars) used for the exercise is referred to as the load. The maximum load that can be lifted a given number of times is called the repetitions maximum (RM). Thus, the figure 6 RM means the greatest weight that can be lifted six times for a given exercise.

## Safety Precautions

The quality of your weight training program will depend to a large extent on the proper performance of the selected exercises. Improper techniques of lifting can result in injury to yourself or to a training partner.

At first when lifting the barbell and weights from the floor to begin an exercise, make sure you lift with the legs and not with the lower back. This is accomplished by placing your feet close to the bar, lowering your hips in a squat position; the head is up and the back is straight. Then lift by straightening the legs. Always check to see that the barbell collars are tight and properly fastened on the bar to prevent the weights from falling. Also when you are lifting a heavy weight load (especially during the bench press, heel lifts, and half squats), be sure you have spotters to assist getting the barbell into position and to remove it when you have completed your set of repetitions. Wear gymwear, especially rubber soled footware to insure stability during the performance of each exercise. In addition, make sure you follow a proper progression for adjusting the weight load. Too heavy a load at the start can cause unnecessary injury. You should finish your workout comfortably tired rather than exhausted.

## Principles and Procedures

An abundance of research has dealt with the most effective ways to train with weights. The recommended principles and procedures that follow are based on conclusions from recent research on college-aged subjects.

Weight training programs that range from 2 RM for one set to 10 RM for three sets all produce significant gains. Dr. Richard Berger, a Temple University researcher in muscular strength and endurance, asserts that the optimal training combination is 6 RM, for three sets, three times a week. Our own experience with weight training programs for young adult men and women supports Berger's conclusion. We feel very confident in recommending the 6 RM, three set, three-day-a-week regimen.

At the beginning of a weight training program, use the barbells with a very light weight load. Learn the correct movements of the various exercises first. Then proceed to add barbell plates (weights) for added resistance. It will take a couple of workout sessions before you establish your 6 RM for each exercise. In general, it is best to start with a moderate amount of resistance and progress from there.

## Exercises

The following exercises comprise only a beginning program for men and women. The recommended training workout takes about 20 minutes of actual lifting. However, the availability of equipment and the time involved in changing the weight loads will lengthen the duration of the workout.

For optimum results keep an accurate record of each workout on a chart like the one shown in Figure 7.1. Record the load and the RM for each exercise. These records will help you accurately regulate your workouts. Remember to increase the load (resistance) after you can easily complete the three sets of six repetitions for a certain load. In addition, it is best to avoid doing the same exercise consecutively. If possible do one set of curls, then bent over rowing, then return to do your second set of curls. Such a pattern will minimize some of the muscular fatigue associated with weight training. Remember the overload is the key to developing strength.

WEIGHT TRAINING RECORD

EXERCISE

| | | 10/4 | 10/6 | 10/8 | 10/11 | 10/13 | 10/15 | 10/18 | | | | | |
|---|---|---|---|---|---|---|---|---|---|---|---|---|---|
| Curl | lb. | 50 | 50 | 50 | 60 | 60 | | | | | | | |
| | RM | 6-6-3 | 6-6-4 | 6-6-6 | 6-5-2 | 6-4-3 | | | | | | | |
| Press | lb. | 60 | 75 | 75 | 75 | 75 | | | | | | | |
| | RM | 6-6-6 | 6-6-4 | 6-6-3 | 6-6-5 | 6-5-5 | | | | | | | |
| Bench Press | lb. | 75 | 75 | 85 | 85 | 85 | | | | | | | |
| | RM | 6-6-4 | 6-6-6 | 6-5-4 | 6-5-4 | 6-5-5 | | | | | | | |
| Upright Rowing | lb. | 60 | 75 | 75 | 75 | 85 | | | | | | | |
| | RM | 6-6-6 | 6-5-4 | 6-5-5 | 6-6-6 | 6-4-2 | | | | | | | |
| Bent–Over Rowing | lb. | 85 | 100 | 100 | 100 | 100 | | | | | | | |
| | RM | 6-6-6 | 6-4-4 | 6-5-5 | 6-5-5 | 6-6-5 | | | | | | | |
| Heel Lifts | lb. | 100 | 125 | 125 | 135 | 135 | | | | | | | |
| | RM | 6-6-6 | 6-6-6 | 6-6-6 | 6-4-4 | 6-4-4 | | | | | | | |
| Half Squats | lb. | 100 | 125 | 125 | 135 | 150 | | | | | | | |
| | RM | 6-6-6 | 6-6-6 | 6-6-6 | 6-6-6 | 6-6-4 | | | | | | | |

*Figure 7.1*

These exercises are commonly used in weight training and conditioning work. Together they are adequate for developing most of the major muscle groups of the body. A warm-up period should precede your weight training routine. Conditioning exercises that involve stretching are needed to loosen the muscles and stimulate the circulation. (See Chapter 5.)

Your beginning load for each exercise has to be determined by trial and error. However, an easy way to approximate it is based on your body weight. Assuming that you are not overweight and that you possess reasonable strength for your age, your body weight corresponds roughly to your strength. Therefore, with each exercise description presented in this chapter, a portion of your body weight is suggested as a beginning load. When you can easily perform more than six reps (on the third set) for a given exercise, then add 5 to 10 pounds or more at your next training session. By following these procedures for three sessions a week, you will experience significant strength gains in six to eight weeks.

Although we all have our own personal preferences, we hope that your program of cardiorespiratory fitness is not neglected or excluded in favor of your weight training program. Weight training programs, when not supplemented with cardiorespiratory training, are not adequate to improving or maintaining a quality fitness level of the heart, lungs, and blood vessels.

## ARM CURLS

| | |
|---|---|
| Purpose: | To develop the flexors of the arms and forearms. |
| Starting Position: | Stand erect, arms fully extended downward, and hold the barbell with an underhand grip (palms out); your hands should be at shoulder-width apart. |
| Movement: | Raise the barbell to your chest by flexing your arms. Your elbows should remain at your sides. If possible, stand erect with your back to a wall. |

Suggested Beginning Load:   One-fourth to one-third of your body weight.

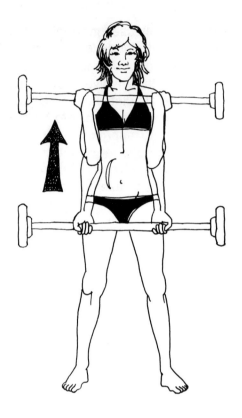

*Arm curls*

## PRESS

| | |
|---|---|
| Purpose: | To develop the extensors of the upper arms and the muscles of the shoulders, back, and upper chest region. |
| Starting Position: | Stand erect. Grasp the barbell with your thumbs pointing inward (overhand grip) and bring it to a resting position on your upper chest with elbows down. |
| Movement: | Push (raise) the bars straight overhead until your arms lock. Then lower the bar back to chest position. |

Suggested Beginning Load:   One-fourth to one-third of your body weight.

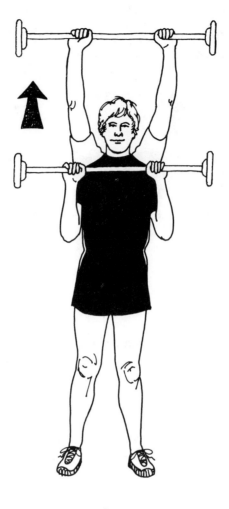

*Press*

## BENCH PRESS*

Purpose:     To develop muscles of the chest and shoulders and the extensors of the arm (triceps).

*Spotters at each end of the barbell are recommended for this exercise.

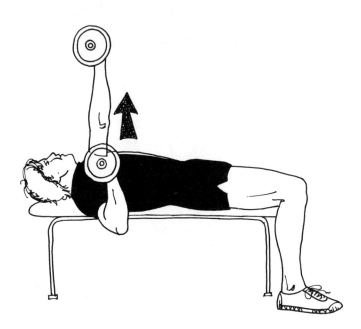

*Bench press*

Starting Position:  Lie on your back on a bench with your knees bent and your feet flat on the floor, straddling the bench. Have a friend hand you the barbell in a position above your chest, with arms up and elbows locked. Your hands should be placed slightly wider than the breadth of your shoulders, thumbs under and down.

Movement:  Lower the barbell to middle of chest and then press it back to the extended position.

Suggested Beginning Load:  One-third to one-half of your body weight.

## UPRIGHT ROWING

Purpose:  To develop the shoulder, back, and arm muscles.

**Starting Position:** Stand erect, arms down. Hold the barbell across your thighs with an overhand grip (thumbs in), hands one to three inches apart.

**Movement:** Raise the bar to a position at shoulder level under your chin. Keep your elbows above the bar throughout the exercise. Return to the starting position.

**Suggested Beginning Load:** One-third to one-half of your body weight.

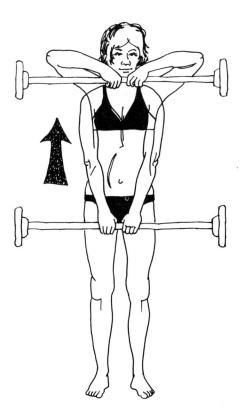

*Upright rowing*

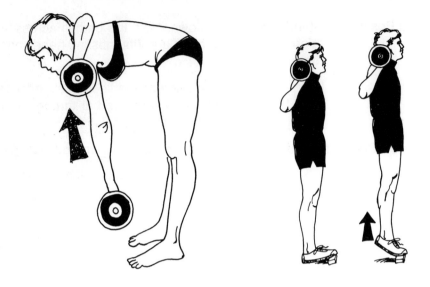

*Bent-over rowing*                    *Heel lifts*

## BENT-OVER ROWING

| | |
|---|---|
| Purpose: | To develop the muscles of the back, back of shoulders, and front of upper arms. |
| Starting Position: | Bend at the waist with your upper body; your back is parallel to the floor and your knees are slightly flexed. Extend your arms downward and grip the barbell with an overhand grip, hands shoulder-width apart. |
| Movement: | Bring the bar directly up to your chest, keeping your back straight and head up. Then return the bar to the extended position (a few inches off of the floor) |
| Suggested Beginning Load: | One-third to one-half of your body weight. |

## HEEL LIFTS*

| | |
|---|---|
| Purpose: | To develop the muscles of the calves and feet. |

*Spotters at each end of the barbell are recommended for this exercise.

Starting Position:     Stand erect with the barbell across your shoulders at the back of your neck. You may use padding on your neck.

Movement:     Raise yourself on your toes to a fully extended position (heels off the floor) and then lower your heels slowly back to the floor. You can get an added range of motion by placing the balls of your feet over a stable two-by-four piece of wood.

Suggested Beginning Load:     One-half to two-thirds of your body weight.

---

## HALF SQUATS*

Purpose:     To develop primarily the muscles of the upper legs.

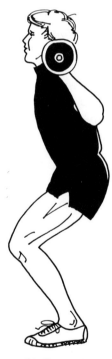

*Half squats*

*Spotters at each end of the barbell are recommended for this exercise.

Starting Position: Stand erect with your feet shoulder-width apart, the barbell resting on your neck, as for heel lifts.

Movement: Lower your body to a semisquating position by bending at the knees. Keep the back straight. Then return to a straight-knee position.

Suggested Beginning Load: One-half to two-thirds of your body weight.

## ISOKINETICS

A new concept of strength building has been emerging in recent years called *isokinetics*. It combines all the advantages of isometrics and isotonics. Briefly, isokinetic exercise involves a maximum effort as in isometric exercise, but the exercise is carried out through a complete range of motion. For developing muscular strength this form of training can place greater demands on the muscle throughout the full range of movement than lifting a barbell. This is the key to isokinetic exercise. Resistance in the muscle throughout the range of isokinetic effort adjusts automatically to the pull or push exerted at any given moment of the exercise. In other words, the amount of resistance created by the muscle always equals the amount of force being applied. This isokinetic-type exercise is now possible because of the development of a new kind of apparatus. You either push or pull against the mechanism, and it resists with the exact force that you apply. An automatic governor mechanism controls not only the resistance but also the speed at which the exercise is done.

Dr. James Counsilman, an outstanding swimming coach from Indiana University, strongly feels that isokinetics exercises are more efficient than other forms of exercise for the development of strength. The one drawback is that the specialized equipment needed for exercising this way cannot be easily obtained. However, with the promise of isokinetic exercise as a sound means for developing strength, it is likely that isokinetic equipment will be less expensive and more readily available for most people in the future. For more detailed information on isokinetics, consult the appropriate readings listed at the end of the chapter.

## KEY WORDS

HYPERTROPHY: The term used to describe the increase in size or mass of a cell, tissue, or organ (e.g., increase in muscle fiber size resulting from strength training).

ISOKINETIC CONTRACTION: A muscle contraction at a constant speed with the muscle generating force against a variable resistance.

ISOMETRIC CONTRACTION: A muscle contraction with the muscle generating force without allowing significant shortening of the muscle (e.g., pushing against a wall).

ISOTONIC CONTRACTION: A muscle contraction with the muscle generating force against a constant resistance with a shortening of the muscle (e.g., curling a barbell).

LOAD: The poundage used for a particular weight training exercise.

MUSCLE FIBER: A structural unit of muscle. Often referred to as muscle cell.

MUSCULAR ENDURANCE: The capacity of a muscle to exert a force repeatedly or to hold a fixed or static contraction over a period of time.

OVERLOAD PRINCIPLE: The physiological fact that a muscle subjected to a greater–than–normal load will increase in size and strength.

POWER: The rate at which force can be produced or the product of force and velocity. Sometimes referred to as the explosive ability to apply force.

REPETITIONS: The number of consecutive contractions performed during each weight training exercise. (See SET.)

REPETITIONS MAXIMUM (RM): The maximum load that can be lifted a given number of times for a particular weight training exercise (e.g., 6 RM refers to the maximum weight that can be performed six times).

SET: The number of bouts performed for each weight training exercise (e.g., three sets of 6 reps). (See REPETITIONS.)

STRENGTH: The capacity of a muscle to exert a force against a resistance.

# SUPPLEMENTARY READINGS

Bender, Jay, Harold Kaplan, and Alex Johnson, "Isometrics—A Critique of Faddism versus Facts." *Journal of Health, Physical Education, and Recreation,* **34**:21, May 1963.

Berger, Richard. "Effect of Varied Weight Training Programs on Strength." *Research Quarterly,* **33**:168, 1962.

Clarke, David H., "Adaptations in Strength and Muscular Endurance Resulting from Exercise." *Exercise and Sports Sciences Reviews,* Vol. 1, Jack H. Wilmore, ed. New York: Academic, 1973.

Clarke, H., *Muscular Strength and Endurance in Man.* Englewood Cliffs, New Jersey: Prentice-Hall, 1966.

Counsilman, James, "Isokinetic Exercise." *Athletic Journal,* **52**:58, February, 1972.

Franz, Edward and Bruce Melin, *Beginning Weight Training.* Belmont, California: Wadsworth, 1965.

Higdon, Hal, "Let's Tell the Truth About Isometrics." *Today's Health,* **43**:58, June, 1965.

Hooks, Gene, *Application of Weight Training to Athletics.* Englewood Cliffs, New Jersey: Prentice-Hall, 1962.

Meisel, Harry J., "Specifistic Exercise." *Swimming World and Junior Swimmer,* **15**:40, January 1974.

O'Shea, John Patrick, *Scientific Principles and Methods of Strength Fitness.* Philadelphia: Addison-Wesley, 1976.

Rosentswieg, Joel and Marilyn Hinson, "Comparing the Three Best Ways of Developing Strength." *Scholastic Coach,* **41**:34, March 1972.

# chapter eight

This chapter presents conditioning methods that are more vigorous and of higher intensity than the previous recommended programs. Continuous training, interval training, and circuit training are forms of training normally engaged in by people who have passed through the normal stages of getting in shape and who now wish to reach a higher level of training. Athletes or people training for specific sports tend to engage in these forms of training.

As you read this chapter give thought to the following statements:

• Interval training involves heavy exercise for a given distance or specified time alternated with light periods of exercise and recovery. It differs from the jog-walk-jog technique because the heavy exercise bouts (such as running) are performed at near-maximal levels.

• Continuous training refers to sustaining an activity for a period of time such as jogging for 30 minutes or cycling for an hour at an intensity approximating your training heart rate.

• Circuit training refers to a specified number of exercise stations that an individual completes in a sequential manner, as quickly as possible, and at a maximal or near maximal intensity. A circuit should promote all-around development.

• As a general rule, the beneficial effects of various endurance-type exercise programs is the same when the total work output performed is the same. However, if you are training for sports that require quick and sudden bursts of movement, you should consider training activities that train the muscle fibers involved in these activities.

# advanced conditioning methods

Prior to this chapter we have presented programs for fitness aimed at a level of intensity that is vigorous, but well short of high-intensity training. Basically the jog-walk-jog and comparable programs of bicycling and swimming are intended to establish general physical fitness, which may be used as a base for sports participation or for more intense training.

The intent of this chapter is to present three types of advanced training: interval, continuous, and circuit. Our cardiorespiratory conditioning programs (as presented earlier) were described as continuous even though periods of recoveries were intermixed with bouts of jogging, cycling, or swimming. The idea behind these programs is to keep the total body moving, recognizing that most people who start out on a fitness program cannot jog continuously for more than 1 to 2 minutes. Thus, a walk or similar rest period is needed. In advanced training, continuous training refers to sustaining a constant tempo for 15 minutes or more. Interval training refers to successive bouts of exercise at near-maximal intensity, alternated with lighter bouts of exercise or in some cases complete rest. In circuit training, on the other hand, exercises are performed at individual stations between which there are no periods of decreased activity. In other words, circuit training is performing all-out.

## INTERVAL TRAINING

Interval training involves heavy exercise for a given distance or a specified time alternated with lighter exercise and recovery. This procedure is repeated. As exercise tolerance permits, the speed of the exercise or the distance covered is increased gradually in the succeeding workouts. It differs from the previous programs presented for cardiorespiratory fitness because the exercise bouts are performed at near-maximal levels of intensity. In other words, the heart rates and energy requirements are greater. More physical pain is associated with this type of training mainly because of the near-maximal efforts that characterize this approach. In general, the pain and discomfort from such training is often associated with more lactate (a metabolic waste product) being produced and accumulated in the muscles.

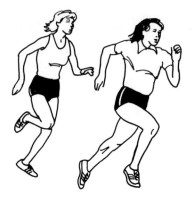

*Interval training refers to successive bouts of exercise at near-maximal intensity, alternated with lighter bouts of exercise.*

Interval training can be an efficient and often time-saving training program. Improvement can be as positive as in any other program probably because the capacity for anaerobic exercise is enhanced. The overload principle is applied and can be regulated to stress the body as severely as one wishes. Each part of the workout is timed and regulated individually, with a definite interval of decreased activity planned between each exercise bout.

Normally, running is a common form of interval training. The overload is regulated by the tempo (speed) of the runs, the amount of time taken during the rest interval, the distance of each running effort, and the number of repetitions. Thus, you can increase the overload by (1) increasing the tempo, (2) decreasing the rest interval, (3) increasing the number of repetitions, and (4) increasing the distance of each run. Changing any one of these regulating factors or changing all of them can increase your exercise workload.

## Setting Up an Interval Training Program

We will use running as the mode of exercise to show you how to set up an interval training program. Your exercise workload will be determined from your present fitness level and your ability to recuperate after each run. Generally, an interval program that emphasizes repetitions or distance and not tempo (pace) is better for beginners. However, for experienced runners or those who wish to improve their running time (e.g., the time to run a mile), a rigid control of the speeds of the runs and of the rest intervals is needed to improve. Training of this type requires a motivated runner who will accept the challenge of the stopwatch and who can tolerate physical discomfort.

In general, the intensity of the exercise bouts should produce near-maximal pulse rates. During the recovery interval the pulse rate should be

## TABLE 8-1   INTERVAL RUNNING CHART

| RECOMMENDED RUNNING SPEEDS | | |
|---|---|---|
| YOUR MILE RUN TIME | 220 YARDS (sec) | 440 YARDS (sec) |
| 4:45- 5:00 | 30-32 | 65- 69 |
| 5:01- 5:15 | 33-34 | 70- 73 |
| 5:16- 5:30 | 35-36 | 74- 77 |
| 5:31- 5:45 | 37-38 | 78- 81 |
| 5:46- 6:00 | 39-40 | 82- 85 |
| 6:01- 6:15 | 41-42 | 86- 89 |
| 6:16- 6:30 | 43-44 | 90- 93 |
| 6:31- 6:45 | 45-46 | 94- 97 |
| 6:46- 7:00 | 47-48 | 98-101 |
| 7:01- 7:15 | 49-50 | 102-105 |
| 7:16- 7:30 | 51-52 | 106-109 |
| 7:31- 7:45 | 53-54 | 110-113 |
| 7:46- 8:00 | 55-56 | 114-117 |
| 8:01- 8:15 | 57-58 | 118-121 |
| 8:16- 8:30 | 59-60 | 122-125 |
| 8:31- 8:45 | 61-62 | 126-129 |
| 8:46- 9:00 | 63-64 | 130-133 |
| 9:01- 9:15 | 65-66 | 134-137 |
| 9:16- 9:30 | 67-68 | 138-141 |
| 9:31- 9:45 | 69-70 | 142-145 |
| 9:46-10:00 | 71-72 | 146-149 |
| 10:01-and up | 73+ | 150 + |

Dosage:

220 yard runs: From 8 to 16 repetitions, with 30 to 45 second rest interval between each run.*

440 yard runs: From 4 to 8 repetitions, with 45 to 60 second rest interval between each run.*

*The time of the rest interval will depend on your pulse rate recovery.

allowed to decrease to between 140 and 120 beats a minute before the exercise bout is repeated. This procedure will greatly increase your endurance capacity.

Table 8.1 presents a progressive overload for your interval running program based on your best time for running a mile. Use of this chart will enable you to improve your running ability for the mile or two-mile run. The distance of each run and the length of the rest interval between runs should be kept constant. In addition, to insure a gradual buildup of fatigue, run each repetition at a pace slightly faster than you can maintain for the mile. On the chart, you can find a suggested time for your runs for either 220- or 440-yard runs. The paces for these distances are slightly faster than your pace for the mile run and you should strive to maintain this speed through all repeated runs. Running a series of repetitions at a constant speed is the key to overloading your cardiorespiratory system to a near-maximal level. The assumption here is that your pulse rate will be near maximal at the end of each run, especially by the third repeat, and your recovery pulse rate will have dropped to between 140 and 120 beats before you begin the next running bout. This chart represents a starting point, and individual differences may require some modification, such as shorter or longer rest intervals or more repetitions.

The same principle for regulating your advanced training bouts for cycling and swimming can be applied; ride or swim at a slightly faster tempo than what you can sustain over a longer distance. For example, if your best time for five miles on a bike is 25 minutes, then you probably should train at a cycling tempo of better than a 5-minute mile—for instance, a 4½- minute mile. Also, if you can swim 300 yards in 10 minutes, then you need to train at a pace faster than 30 yards per minute. So 25 yards a minute with a rest of 30 to 60 seconds are reasonable beginning times for an interval program. Again, individual differences make it unwise to develop "cook-book" type programs to meet all possibilities. Instead, application of the basic guidelines of overload, such as presented here and in Chapter Four, is more practical.

## CONTINUOUS TRAINING

Many exercise programs and most sports are generally intermittent, that is, short periods of activity interrupted by periods of rest or very light work. Nevertheless, physical fitness training for the average person generally follows a continuous pattern. Especially after the beginning stages, a level of training is reached where the activity can be sustained for longer than 10

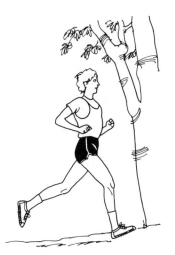

*Continuous training refers to sustaining a constant tempo for 15 minutes or more.*

minutes. In our experience as soon as a man or woman gets to the point in their training where they can sustain a mile or more of jogging, they very seldom return to intermittent- or interval-type training. As previously mentioned, unless you are training for high level competition requiring both aerobic and anaerobic capacities, continuous training appears to be an adequate means for reaching your optimal cardiorespiratory or aerobic fitness level. Once accustomed to continuous jogging, cycling, or swimming you can easily provide a sufficient stimulus to your heart, lungs, and muscles during the recommended 30-minute exercise period.

In fact, once you can sustain continuous exercise for more than 30 minutes, it becomes much easier to continue for 45 minutes or more. Generally, at this stage in your fitness development, local muscular fatigue (tired leg muscles) becomes more of a limiting factor than the cardiorespiratory components. Furthermore, being able to sustain your chosen mode of continuous exercise for a given period of time makes it easier to estimate your caloric expenditure for that particular workout. (See Chapter 9 for ways of estimating the caloric costs of various physical activities.)

## CONTINUOUS VERSUS INTERVAL TRAINING

The main goals in cardiorespiratory training are improving the capacity of the central circulation (heart and lungs) and increasing the capacity of the exercising muscles to use oxygen. This capacity to consume oxygen at your maximal ability is called your aerobic capacity, and is recognized as a functional measure of your cardiorespiratory fitness. The relative magnitude and duration of the exercise movements during the training session provides the stimulus for developing your aerobic fitness. A question often asked is whether interval training is superior to continuous training for developing one's aerobic capacity. Many writers on athletic training are convinced that interval training is the best form of training for improvement of endurance capacity. In contrast, other studies have failed to demonstrate any real differences. In fact, there is convincing evidence that when the total work output performed is the same for both training methods, the improvement is the same. Dr. Bengt Saltin, a Scandinavian exercise physiologist, in a recent review stated that interval training does not appear to have an advantage over continuous training in enhancing endurance capacity (aerobic capacity) when total work output is approximately the same. For that matter, he finds that neither is continuous training better than discontinuous (interval), and he recommends using both forms of training interchangeably for high performance conditioning. However, Dr. Saltin does suggest the possibility that interval training, because it requires that very intense efforts be repeated, may be preferable for developing the higher <u>anaerobic</u> capacities[1] that are so necessary in top level sports performance.

His theory is based on biochemical studies of muscle fibers. Human muscle is composed of two types of fibers, slow twitch and fast twitch. The <u>slow twitch fiber</u> has a higher overall capacity to use oxygen for energy than the fast twitch fibers. Conversely, the <u>fast twitch fibers</u> have a higher anaerobic potential than slow twitch fibers. However, the oxidative capacity (aerobic) of both fiber types can be increased by physical training. Additional biochemical studies have shown that the slow twitch fiber is recruited more readily during prolonged endurance work (continuous) where its oxidative potential can be fully utilized. In contrast, fast twitch fibers appear to be more suited to high speed intense work of short duration (interval). In other words, fast twitch muscle cells are first used in short sudden bursts of activity. Training studies have indicated that *both* slow and fast twitch fibers are recruited during interval training whereas during continuous work, the involvement of the fast twitch fibers is not as readily noticeable.

In summary, the key factor to remember is that during continuous exer-

---

[1]Anaerobic refers to energy used by the contractile apparatus of the muscle fiber that does not depend on an immediate source of oxygen. (For a more complete explanation see Chapter Two.)

cise the nervous system tends only to use the slow twitch fiber, but during repeated short efforts the fast twitch fibers are used more readily. Thus, if you are training for sports that require quick movements, for example, tennis, karate, and handball, you need to train the fast twitch as well as the slow twitch fibers. In these situations you should consider some workouts using interval training methods. If your concern is in only improving your aerobic capacity (cardiorespiratory fitness), then a continuous program will provide a sufficient stimulus for optimal training. Remember, both types of training (continuous or interval) can enhance your endurance capacity.

## CIRCUIT TRAINING

Circuit training was developed in Great Britain as a systematic and progressive conditioning program that would appeal to young people. It is designed to provide a vigorous, all-around workout over a short period of time. Specifically, circuit training aims at developing muscular strength and endurance, flexibility, cardiorespiratory endurance, and, in some instances,

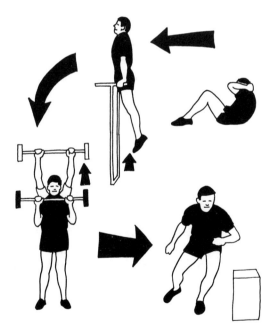

*Circuit training refers to completing a specified number of exercise stations as quickly as possible.*

coordination. Such elements as running, calisthenics, and weight training can all be incorporated into the program.

A *circuit* is a specified number of exercise stations that are consecutively arranged in a given area. Each individual participant faces the challenge of completing the entire circuit as quickly as possible. Circuit training differs from other fitness programs in that the activities are all performed at a maximal or near-maximal level over a time period ranging from 10 to 20 minutes. In recent years athletic coaches have recognized the worth of such a program and have utilized the circuit training method for conditioning their squads. The near-maximal overload on a variety of activities, geared to one's abilities, makes circuit training one of the best ways for developing all-around physical fitness.

## Setting Up a Circuit

In setting up your circuit, choose activities that are feasible and use care in planning your stations. Remember, *a circuit should promote all-around development.* A variety of selected exercises for muscular strength and endurance, flexibility, athletic skill, and cardiorespiratory endurance will provide a complete workout in a limited time. At the same time, however, you can emphasize any particular traits you wish to develop by including the appropriate activities. Before you set up a circuit of stations you should decide whether there are any fitness traits you wish to stress. For example, you may wish to strengthen the upper arm and shoulder area for your tennis game. Thus, you might include several exercises that strengthen these muscles—for example, pull-ups, push-ups, or weight training exercises such as the arm curl and press. For cardiorespiratory fitness you can include jogging and, in some cases, even swimming or cycling as part of your circuit.

Any number of facilities can be used for circuit training: gymnasiums, outdoor playgrounds, athletic fields, swimming pools, a lake, parking lots, or even hallways. Ideally, your school or university may have permanent equipment, such as pull-up bars, sit-up areas, and obstacle courses that are suited for circuit training. Nevertheless, no matter what your situation is, with a little creativity it is possible to set up a functional circuit. Though any circuit is dependent on the facilities available and the objectives desired, the program suggested in Table 8.2 may serve as a model for setting up your own circuit.

First, the stations should be arranged so that similar activities, using the same muscle groups, do not follow one another. If you are in a situation

## TABLE 8.2

| STATION | EXERCISE DOSAGE |
|---|---|
| 1. Run | 2 laps* |
| 2. Pull-ups | 4 reps |
| 3. Repeated vertical jumps (two-hand touch) | 10 reps† |
| 4. Sit-ups (bent knee) | 25 reps |
| 5. Press (barbell, 30 to 40 lb) | 10 reps |
| 6. Run | 3 laps |
| 7. Leg-overs (each side) | 5 reps |
| 8. Bench stepping (bleacher) | 30 steps |
| 9. Squat thrusts | 6 reps |
| 10. Bent-over rowing (barbell, 30 to 40 lb.) | 10 reps |
| 11. Agility run | 4 reps |
| 12. Opposite toe touching | 10 reps |
| 13. Upright rowing (barbell, 20 lb) | 6 to 10 reps |
| 14. Run | 3 laps |

*A running lap is equivalent to 110 yards.

†Generally horizontal lines (tape) are placed on a wall at 7, 8, 9 feet intervals as targets to jump for.

where a permanent circuit is set up, a numbered sign at each station generally designates the activity to be performed. You can determine the amount of work to be performed at each station with preliminary testing at the selected stations. For example, if you test yourself on pull-ups and find you can do a maximum of six, then we suggest that you halve this number and set the exercise load at the pull-up station at three. This same procedure can be carried out with the other exercises. In some cases, such as bench stepping, you may wish to select a work load equal to about 30 to 60 seconds of exercise.

Usually you should repeat the circuit after a two- to three-minute rest. Record the time it takes to complete the circuit. Your improvement will become apparent as the time required for you to complete the circuit is decreased. Generally we recommend a 10 to 15-station circuit, requiring from 8 to 12 minutes to complete. When you have made significant improvement (generally a reduction in time of 3 to 4 minutes), retest yourself and increase the number of repetitions.

Additional exercises are described in Chapters 5 and 7. (See the index for individual exercises.) We suggest you make a list of your sequence of stations indicating the amount of laps, or reps you wish to complete at each station. Some stations might include a rope climb, running up bleacher steps, hand-walking a horizontal ladder, tumbling exercises, parallel-bar hand walking, and obstacle climbing, crawling, or dodging. If you are outside, a swim in a pool or lake could even be incorporated. Depending on the facilities available and your desired objectives, the circuit training method offers limitless opportunities for beneficial conditioning.

The advantages of circuit training are many. (1) Circuit training allows each subject to progress at his or her own prescribed rate of work. (2) It provides an opportunity for vigorous overall development in a very short period of time. (3) It assures progressive overload in an organized manner. (4) Each individual can anticipate some degree of success.

With a little imagination, circuit training can become an excellent addition to a well-balanced program of sports and physical fitness. However, because of its "near maximal" nature, extreme caution should be taken when beginning a circuit training program. Preliminary conditioning according to the guidelines presented in previous chapters is a wise step, in order to prevent unnecessary injury or any other possible harmful incidents. In general, circuit training is not recommended for older people, especially for untrained, sedentary people. It is a form of high intensity training that can provide all-around development.

## KEY WORDS

ANAEROBIC: Means "without oxygen" and refers to the output of energy for muscular contraction when the oxygen supply is insufficient.

CIRCUIT TRAINING: A routine of selected exercises or activities performed in sequence at individual stations, as rapidly as possible.

CONTINUOUS TRAINING: Sustaining a constant tempo of exercise for a period of time. In beginning programs, bouts of brisk walking are generally alternated with short bouts of exercise.

FAST TWITCH MUSCLE FIBER: A type of muscle fiber with "fast" contractile characteristics that has a low capacity to use oxygen. These fibers are the first to be used in short sudden bursts of activities (See SLOW TWITCH MUSCLE FIBER).

INTERVAL TRAINING: Successive bouts of exercise at near-maximal intensity alternated with lighter periods of rest or exercise such as brisk walking.

SLOW TWITCH MUSCLE FIBER: A type of muscle fiber with "slow" contractile characteristics that has a high capacity to use oxygen. These fibers are those used primarily during endurance type activities such as jogging, swimming, and cycling.

## SUPPLEMENTARY READINGS

Annarino, Anthony, *Developmental Conditioning For Physical Education and Athletics.* St. Louis: Mosby, 1972.

Berger, Richard, *Conditioning For Men.* Boston: Allyn and Bacon, 1973.

Costill, David L., *What Research Tells the Coach About Distance Running.* Washington, D. C.: American Alliance for Health, Physical Education and Recreation, 1968.

Daniels, Jack, Robert Fitts, and George Sheehan, *Conditioning for Distance Running.* New York: John Wiley & Sons, 1978.

Faulkner, John A., *What Research Tells the Coach About Swimming.* Washington, D.C.: American Alliance for Physical Education and Recreation, 1967.

Fox, Edward L. and Donald K. Mathews, *Interval Training.* Philadelphia: Saunders, 1974.

Henderson, Joe, *Jog, Run, Race.* Mountain View, California: World Publications, 1977.

Howell, Maxwell L. and W. R. Morford, "Circuit Training for a College Fitness Program." *Journal of Health, Physical Education and Recreation,* **25** :30, 1964.

Johnson, Perry and Donald Stolberg, *Conditioning.* Englewood Cliffs, New Jersey: Prentice-Hall, 1971.

Morgan, R. E. and G. T. Adamson, *Circuit Training.* Second edition, London: Bell and Sons, 1961.

Sorani, Robert, *Circuit Training.* Dubuque: Brown, 1966.

Wilmore, Jack H., *Athletic Training and Physical Fitness: Physiological Principles & Practices of the Conditioning Process.* Boston: Allyn and Bacon, 1976.

# PART THREE

# ADDITIONAL CONCERNS RELATED TO PHYSICAL FITNESS

# chapter nine

In this chapter the interrelationship of nutrition and exercise is explored as a basis for sound weight control. Much has been written about diets and weight control through exercise, and much of it lacks any scientific basis. The essential facts of nutrition and related information concerning exercise are presented here so that you can make sensible decisions.

The role of each nutrient is discussed along with the basics for a nutritious diet. Seven food groups are utilized instead of the four groups commonly used. The caloric values for a variety of foods are presented and a means for calculating your daily energy needs is also provided.

The remainder of the chapter deals with the role of exercise as a means to better control of body weight. Details concerning the relative energy costs (Calories) in a variety of conditioning and sports activities are presented. In addition, some common misconceptions about exercise and weight control are discussed.

As you read this chapter give thought to the following statements:

• The principle that your energy intake (food) and energy output (physical activity) must be kept in balance is easy to understand but the real problem for many people is to control this balance.

• Proteins represent the basic structural substance of the body; carbohydrates are the primary energy foods; and fat is also an energy food but one not readily burned off by inactive people.

• Your daily energy needs depend on such factors as body size, age, and the type and amount of your daily physical activity.

• In determining your ideal weight, how fat you are is more important than how much you weigh. Determining the proportion of fat tissue in your body rather than scale weight is a better indicator for estimating your proper weight.

• The term MET refers to the rate of energy expended: one MET is equivalent to the energy needed at rest. Four METS depicts energy requirements four times greater than rest, which is representative of low to moderate exercise. (Activities requiring eight to twelve

# nutrition, weight control, and exercise

METS would be classified as vigorous.)

• Whether one walks or jogs a specified distance, the number of calories required to complete the distance would be approximately the same.

• Research does not support the theory that if you exercise a spot or area of your body, you will reduce the excess fat in that region. Instead, loss of fat tends to be uniform in proportion to the amount present at any given site. Thus, for fat reduction, total body movement activities that can be sustained over a period have shown to be the best.

• The practice of dehydrating (losing water) is a useless and dangerous means for weight loss.

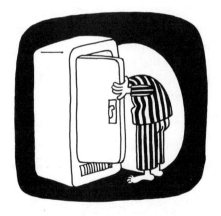

*When you eat more than your daily energy needs, the excess energy is stored as body fat.*

In recent years the interest in diets and weight control has increased. In fact, the shelves of newsstands and bookstores are constantly being deluged with publications dealing with nutrition and weight control. At the same time, the food industry continues to offer new products and new ways to prepare food. We constantly worry about what to eat and what not to eat.

In addition, advertisements frequently promote the "fast" or "easy way" to rid the body of excess fat. Quite often such claims are sheer nonsense and lack any scientific basis. The purpose of this chapter is to explain the essential facts of nutrition and their relation to weight control and exercise, so that these claims can be evaluated wisely.

The basic principle of weight control is quite simple. However, for many people, the ability to control their body weight has met with limited success. Fundamentally, your energy intake (food) and energy output (physical activity) must be kept in balance. When you eat more than your daily energy needs, the excess energy is stored as body fat. When you eat less, you burn stored fat for energy. Understanding this principle is no problem. The real problem is to control creeping overweight and the associated health problems that are so common in our society today. Regular exercise coupled with sound eating habits offer a sensible approach for keeping off excess body fat.

## NUTRITION BASICS

Nutrition is the study of the food we eat and how the body uses it. Foods provide us with a wide variety of necessary substances, or nutrients. These substances are essential for building and repairing the body, and for providing the energy needed for efficient functioning. Energy is provided by three basic classes of nutrients in the food we eat: proteins, carbohydrates, and fats. Minerals, vitamins, and water are also essential for life. Here is a brief summary of the role of each nutrient.

### Protein

All life requires protein. It is the basic structural substance of each cell in the body. Protein provides structure to bones, skin, muscle fibers, and many

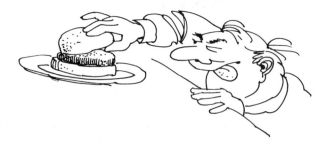

*Nutrition is a study of the food we eat and how the body uses it.*

tissues. It is the source of enzymes and hormones, which control and regulate chemical reactions in our bodies. Specialized proteins are also present in blood in the form of clotting agents and oxygen-carrying molecules. When we eat, these basic building blocks in the food are broken down into amino acids. These amino acids are then built up again in various parts of the body into formations such as those described above (e.g., cell membrane, enzymes, etc.). The major sources of protein come from foods of animal origin: meat, fish, poultry, eggs, and milk. Nutritionists also suggest peas, beans, and nuts as good substitutes for animal protein. Your daily diet should be at least 15 percent protein.

## Carbohydrates

Carbohydrates (starches and sugars) provide us with energy and fuel for performing bodily functions, such as forming new chemical compounds, transmitting nerve impulses, and supplying the primary energy for vigorous muscular activity. (In contrast, proteins are not used significantly for energy during physical activity.) Good sources of starches are potatoes, beans, peas, grains (e.g., wheat, oats, corn, and rice), flour, macaroni, spaghetti, noodles, grits, bread, cakes, and breakfast cereal. Sweets such as candy, jams, jellies, table sugar, honey, molasses, and concentrated syrups provide sugars. Fruits, vegetables, and fruit juices also contain carbohydrates.

Currently there is much confusion concerning the eating of sugar, a carbohydrate, and its possible adverse affects on the body. Doesn't the body need sugar? The answer is yes, but our bodies do not need to ingest table sugar, which is refined sugar. Quite often the terms table sugar (sucrose) and blood sugar (glucose) are used interchangeably. However, they are quite different and this confusion leads to much misunderstanding.

There are many forms of carbohydrates such as lactose, a sugar found in milk, fructose, a fruit sugar, and starches. Starch is found in corn and various grains from which bread, cereal, spaghetti, and pastries are made. Also, large amounts of starch are present in beans, peas, and potatoes. All these forms of sugar serve the same basic purpose: to provide glucose for the body. The key point, however, is that the milk sugars, fruit sugars, and starches supply us with other needed nutrients—they do more than satisfy our "sweet tooth." They provide many of the essential minerals and vitamins needed in a balanced diet.

Many nutritionists feel the overeating of sugar (the stuff you put in coffee and on your cereal) and especially the refined sugars found in many processed foods are, in a large part, responsible for a number of dangerous diseases. Obesity, heart disease, and adult-onset diabetes have been linked with overconsumption of sugar. Also, it is well established that tooth decay is related to eating sugar-based foods.

Sugar must be consumed in moderation and not to the exclusion of other important foods in your diet. The problem with sugar-based foods is that they taste so good and we want to eat too much of them. It has been estimated that the average American consumes well over 100 pounds of refined sugar per year. Much of these sugars are hidden in the processed foods that we consume regularly, which are called "empty calorie" foods because they provide nothing but energy. It seems wise to cut down on sugar intake by avoiding sweet snacks and foods high in sugar content. In other words, select foods that provide a good nutrient return for the caloric investment.

The human body requires certain amounts of all the nutrients and since the typical American diet contains 25 percent or more of its calories as sugar, the Senate Select Committee on Nutrition and Human Needs has recently (1977) recommended cutting your intake of sugar (sucrose) to about 15 percent of your total calories. The overeating of sugars may rob our bodies of the necessary vitamins and minerals that result from a well-balanced diet. The more refined sugar you can eliminate from your daily eating, the better. Nutritionist Dr. Jean Mayer sums it up well: "About the only good thing I can say for sugar is that it tastes good!"

Approximately 55 percent of the food you eat should be in the form of carbohydrate. With this in mind, the above recommendation from the Senate Committee infers that 40 percent of your total calories should be carbohydrates other than sugar. This means eating more vegetables, fruits, and starches. In addition, whenever you take in more carbohydrates than your body needs, the excess is converted to fat and stored. Hence, a person who eats an excess of carbohydrates (excess calories) increases the body's fat content, which may eventually lead to obesity.

## Fats

The main components of fats, <u>fatty acids</u>, are a concentrated source of energy. Weight for weight, fats provide more than twice as much energy (calories) as either carbohydrates or protein. <u>Fat</u> is a necessary nutrient. Besides being an important part of the cell structure, fat acts as an insulator and protector of vital parts of the body, and it provides additional energy for muscular activity. Common sources of fats are bacon and fatty meats, butter, margarine, shortening, cooking and salad oils, cream, most cheeses, mayonnaise, nuts, milk, eggs, and chocolate. Of course, anything cooked in fat will contain fat.

Not all fats are alike. There are two types of fats: saturated and unsaturated. Saturated fats come from meat, whole milk, cheese, and butter. This type of fat does not melt at room temperature. In contrast, unsaturated fats tend to be in a liquid form at room temperature. Saturated fats are known to raise levels of cholesterol in the bloodstream. Because of this, many nutritionists and physicians are trying to persuade people to reduce the saturated fats in their diet. Your diet should be about 30 percent fat, but it is recommended that you replace *some* of the saturated fat in the diet with unsaturated or polyunsaturated fats. Unsaturated fats are found in peanut and olive oils. Polyunsaturated fats are found in corn, soybean, cottonseed, and, particularly, safflower oils. A recent report of a national nutrition committee recommends reducing your saturated fat consumption to about 10 percent of your total energy intake and balance that with polyunsaturated fats (20 percent). It is believed that if you reduce your intake of solid fats to a minimum and use unsaturated or polyunsaturated fats as an alternative to animal fat, you will lower the levels of serum blood cholesterol.

Cholesterol, a fatty-like substance, is found only in animal products, especially egg yolks, liver, and brain and in shrimp, lobster, and other crustacean foods. Cholesterol is necessary in the body, and your body is capable of producing what it needs. It is required for many of the complex functions of the body and is used in making the important sex hormones. When there is too much of it, however, it tends to settle in the walls of the blood vessels and can impair circulation. (For more information on cholesterol and its relationship to heart disease, see Chapter 10, "Activity and Heart Disease.")

## Minerals
Many minerals are required by the body. They give strength and rigidity to certain body tissues and assist with numerous vital functions. Calcium, iodine, iron, phosphorous, magnesium, and others are vitally important to the functioning of body systems. For example, calcium is the most abundant mineral in the body and combines with phosphorus to form the teeth and bones. Calcium is also crucial for normal functioning of muscles. Phosphorus is an essential component for supplying energy to the body. Iodine is an important ingredient in thyroxin, a hormone that governs the rate of energy metabolism in the body. Iron is a key component of hemoglobin in the blood.

Sodium and potassium are also minerals. They play a key role in controlling and regulating fluid balance in the body. These elements, called electrolytes, are present mainly in the fluids inside and surrounding the cells and they are essential for proper transmission of nerve impulses. Sodium is present in all living matter such as meats, poultry, fish, and vegetables. It is added in the processing of food as preservatives, stabilizers, and additives. Table salt is a spice that contains sodium. It is well-known by the medical profession that the origin of high blood pressure is related to the amounts of salts eaten or, more precisely, the sodium ingested by the individual. (For more information on high blood pressure, see Chapter 10, "Activity and Heart Disease.) Medical doctors strongly recommend limiting your sodium ingestion by not salting food and avoiding products containing sodium additives. A recent decision by baby food processors to no longer add salt to their products demonstrates national awareness of the dangers of an excess of salt in the diet.

As a general rule, eating balanced meals by following recommended allotments of the seven basic foods—presented later in this chapter—will provide you with your daily needs for minerals.

**Vitamins**
Vitamins are organic substances needed in small amounts by the body and essential for the proper functioning of muscles and nerves. They also play a dynamic role in releasing energy from foods and in promoting normal growth of body tissues. The cells of the body cannot form these substances and therefore the vitamin needs of the body must be provided by the food you eat.

Some vitamins tend to be retained within the body and stored in fat, whereas many vitamins are transported in the fluids of the tissues and cells and are not stored. These vitamins must be consumed in the daily diet. Any excessive ingestion of these vitamins is usually excreted in the urine on a daily basis. Thus, ingesting more vitamins than recommended will be of limited or no benefit. All the required vitamins can be found in a well-rounded nutritious diet. Only in rare cases do healthy people who eat well-balanced meals require vitamin supplements.

**Water**
The body's need for water exceeds its need for food. About 60 percent of your body is water, and water is second only to oxygen in importance. Water provides the medium (body fluids) for transporting nutrients and

hormones throughout the body and for removing wastes from the body. Water also plays a vital role in regulating body temperature. You get the water you need not only by drinking it directly but from the foods you eat.

## NATIONAL DIETARY GOALS

The growing recognition of the importance of nutrition in health has led to a need for basic goals and practical guides for an individual to follow. A Committee on Nutrition and Human Needs in 1977 published a report focusing on the health concerns related to the eating patterns of the average American. After considering many scientific concerns, this group recommended some dietary goals. This report generated widespread interest and controversy. It stated that the composition of our diet has changed radically in recent years. For example, the complex carbohydrates (fruit, vegetables, and grain products), previously the mainstay of the diet, have now been replaced by increased consumption of fat and refined sugars. These changes are regarded as detrimental to overall health. That is, this overconsumption of fat and sugar, along with increased ingestion of cholesterol, salt, and alcohol, has been related to six of the ten leading causes of death in the United States.

This report recommends six dietary goals that represent "prudent" eating habits and seven guidelines for changes in food selection and preparation. The following guidelines were listed: to avoid overweight, consume only as much energy (Calories) as is expended; if overweight, decrease energy intake and increase energy expenditure (which is the theme of this chapter). Increase the eating of complex carbohydrates (naturally occurring sugars such as fruits, vegetables, grains); decrease the consumption of refined and processed sugars to about 10 percent of your total energy intake; reduce the overall consumption of fat to about 30 percent of your energy intake; reduce saturated fat consumption to 10 percent and balance that with polyunsaturated (liquid) fats; reduce cholesterol consumption to about 300 mg a day; and limit the intake of sodium by reducing the intake of salt to about 5 grams a day.

If we accept these guidelines, then the following adjustments in food selection and preparation must be incorporated into our daily eating habits; increase consumption of fruits, vegetables, and whole grain products; decrease consumption of refined and other processed sugars and foods high in such sugars; decrease consumption of foods high in total fat and replace with fats obtained from vegetable sources (polyunsaturated); decrease consumption of animal fat by choosing meats, poultry, and fish with low amounts of saturated fat; substitute low fat and nonfat milk for whole milk and low fat dairy products for high fat dairy products; decrease consumption of butterfat, eggs, and other high cholesterol sources; decrease the consumption of salt and foods high in salt content.

It is important to note that the committee recognizes that these dietary recommendations do not guarantee protection from the killer diseases; they do, however, increase the probability of improved protection.

In summary, these guidelines have been suggested to assist you in making wise food choices that are consistent with good health. The combination of sound nutrition and a vigorous and regular stimulus of the total body (jogging, swimming, cycling) can lead to a life-style of quality living.

## BASICS FOR A NUTRITIOUS DIET

Food provides our bodies with the necessary nutrients for efficient functioning. A sound nutritional diet must be balanced with a variety of foods. In recent years, nutritionists have tended to divide all foods into four basic groups. However, Dr. Jean Mayer, former Professor of Nutrition at Harvard and world-famous scientist, has challenged the shortcomings of this classification and proposed a return to the seven food groups. For example, he considers it absurd to classify all fruits and vegetables together; nutritionally there are many basic differences among them. In accordance with Dr. Mayer's suggestions, the seven basic food groups are presented here, along with daily recommendations for a sound nutritional diet.

### The Seven Food Groups

#### Milk and Milk Products. (At Least Two Servings Daily.)
This group meets the requirements for calcium; it contributes vitamins $B_2$, $B_{12}$, and A, a large number of minerals (iron not included), and high-quality protein. Low-fat milk, if fortified with vitamin D, may be substituted for whole milk. Cheese, yogurt, cottage cheese, and ice cream also belong in this group.

#### Bread, Cereals, and Pasta. (At least Two Servings Daily.)
This group helps fill the body's energy needs with carbohydrates; protein, the B vitamins, and iron are also found in this group; vitamin E is found in wheat germ.

### Meat, Poultry, Fish, Eggs, Dried Beans, and Nuts. (At Least Two Servings Daily.)

All these foods provide large amounts of protein. Poultry and fish are lower in fat than most meats; eggs are rich in practically all vitamins and minerals, but high in cholesterol; liver is also high in cholesterol, but a good source for iron and vitamin A; vegetable proteins (such as soybeans) are also adequate protein foods.

### Butter and Fortified Margarine. (At Least One Serving Daily.)

These foods contribute vitamin A and lots of calories. Butter, an animal fat, should be avoided by those with cholesterol problems; margarines high in polyunsaturated oils (such as corn or safflower oil) are good butter substitutes if fortified with vitamin A.

### Green, Yellow, and Leafy Vegetables. (At Least One Serving Daily.)

These are good sources of vitamins A, E, the B vitamins, and minerals. Spinach, turnip, carrots, pumpkin, and squash are good choices for this food group.

### Citrus Fruits, Tomatoes, Raw Cabbage, and Salad Greens. (At Least One Serving Daily.)

Vitamin C is the essential nutrient found in this group. This vitamin, because it cannot be stored, must be replenished daily in the body. Salad greens, such as lettuce and cabbage are not as high in vitamin C as are the citrus fruits (oranges, grapefruits, tangerines) and tomatoes.

### Potatoes, Other Vegetables, and Fruits. (At Least One Serving Daily.)

This group provides various amounts of vitamin C, minerals, some protein, and energy for the body's needs; potatoes, broccoli, green peppers, and cauliflower are important vegetables in this group; high-nutrition fruits include berries, cherries, melons, and peaches.

With these guidelines it is not necessary to spend a great deal of time worrying about whether the food you eat is good for you. Many foods contain the elements you need for good health. To insure a well-balanced diet, be sure to eat a wide variety of foods. Selections from each of the seven food groups, in moderation, is the best plan for balanced daily eating.

## Caloric Values of Food

All the energy released from food eventually becomes heat in the body. The rate of heat production in the body depends on the energy released from the foods ingested. Energy expenditure in the body and potential energy in foods are measured in Calories.

Table 9.1 gives a caloric equivalent chart for selected foods. A more detailed summary of the nutritional value of foods can be found in *Nutritive Value of Foods,* United States Department of Agriculture, Bulletin No. 72 (Washington D.C.: U.S. Government Printing Office, 1970). This chart of calorie values will assist you in formulating either a weight-loss diet or a weight-maintenance diet. The portions listed in the table are servings of reasonable size.

## Determining Your Energy Needs

The energy needs of the body depend on factors such as body size, age, and the type and amount of your daily physical activity. Your basal metabolic rate (BMR) and caloric expenditure in normal daily activities combine to represent your required energy needs. *Basal metabolism* refers to the minimal rate of energy required to maintain the life processes of the body at complete rest. This figure is determined by measuring the amount of oxygen consumed during a period of time you are relaxed, lying at complete rest, and without food for at least 12 hours.

The oxygen used by your body goes to release the energy in food. Therefore, oxygen uptake denotes the amount of the energy the body utilizes. Most authorities set the basal oxygen requirement of the body at 3.5 milliliters per kilogram of body weight per minute. For a man weighing 70 kilograms this rate is equivalent to 245 milliliters of oxygen per minute, or a basal metabolic rate of 14.7 liters of oxygen per hour. If we multiply the basal metabolic rate by the resting energy equivalent of one liter of oxygen, 4.8 Calories, we can calculate the total quantity of energy liberated within the body during the hour. That figure turns out to be 70.56 Calories. For 24 hours this works out as 1693 Calories.

When the BMR is calculated for other body weights, we find that one kilogram (2.2 lb) of body weight burns approximately one Calorie per hour. Based on this premise, and knowing your weight in kilograms you can set a rough estimate of your basal metabolic rate for 24 hours. A 77-kilogram (170-lb) man, for example, would use 77 Calories per hour, or about 1848 Calories per day. To check the accuracy of this figure, we can calculate it in another way. Using a basal metabolic rate of 3.5 mililiters of oxygen per

# TABLE 9.1 A CALORIC EQUIVALENT CHART

| FOOD DESCRIPTION | SERVING SIZE | APPROXIMATE CALORIES |
|---|---|---|
| **BEVERAGES** | | |
| Beer | 12 oz. | 150 |
| Cola (carbonated) | 12 oz. | 150 |
| Milk (whole) | 12 oz. | 240 |
| Milk (skim) | 12 oz. | 135 |
| Lemonade | 12 oz. | 165 |
| Soft Drinks (carbonated) | 12 oz. | 150 |
| Tea (no cream or sugar) | | 0 |
| | | |
| **BREADS AND CRACKERS** | | |
| Blueberry muffin | one 2½" dia. | 140 |
| Frankfurter or hamburger bun | one bun | 120 |
| Hard roll | one aver. size | 155 |
| White bread | one slice | 65 |
| Doughnut (plain) | 1 aver. size | 200 |
| Cracker | 1 small round | 18 |
| | | |
| **CEREALS AND GRAIN PRODUCTS** | | |
| Bran Flakes | 1 cup | 105 |
| Corn Flakes | 1 cup | 100 |
| Macaroni (cooked) | 1 cup | 190 |
| Oatmeal (cooked) | 1 cup | 130 |
| Pancakes | 1 cake 4" dia. | 60 |
| Rice (cooked) | 1 cup | 225 |
| Spaghetti (cooked) | 1 cup | 155 |
| | | |
| **MEATS** | | |
| *Beef* | | |
| Hamburger Patty (lean ground) | 4 oz. | 245 |
| Hamburger patty (regular) | 4 oz. | 325 |
| Roast Beef | 4 oz. | 220 |
| Steak, broiled, sirloin | 4 oz. | 440 |
| *Pork* | | |
| Bacon | 2 slices | 90 |
| Chops, lean | 4 oz. | 300 |
| Ham, baked | 4 oz. | 325 |
| *Sausages* | | |
| Bologna | 2 slices 3" dia. | 80 |
| Frankfurter | 2 oz. | 170 |

TABLE 9.1 *(continued)*

| FOOD DESCRIPTION | SERVING SIZE | APPROXIMATE CALORIES |
|---|---|---|
| **EGGS, CHEESE, CREAM** | | |
| Coffee cream | 1 tbsp | 30 |
| Cottage cheese (creamed) | 4 oz | 132 |
| Cottage cheese (uncreamed) | 4 oz | 84 |
| Egg, fried or scrambled w/fat | 1 medium | 110 |
| Egg, soft or poached | 1 medium | 78 |
| Process American cheese | 1 oz | 80 |
| Whipping cream | 1 tbsp | 55 |
| **POULTRY** | | |
| Chicken, all meat (broiled) | 4 oz | 150 |
| Chicken (fried) | 1/2 breast | 155 |
| Turkey (roasted) | 4 oz | 220 |
| **SOUPS** | | |
| Beef noodle (with water) | 1 cup | 70 |
| Cream of chicken (with milk) | 1 cup | 180 |
| Split pea (with water) | 1 cup | 145 |
| Tomato (with water) | 1 cup | 90 |
| Tomato (with milk) | 1 cup | 175 |
| Vegetable beef (with water) | 1 cup | 80 |
| **SPREADS AND SUGARS** | | |
| Chocolate syrup | 1 fluid oz | 90 |
| Granulated sugar | 1 tbsp | 48 |
| Honey | 1 tbsp | 65 |
| Jams, marmalades | 1 tbsp | 55 |
| Maple syrup | 1 tbsp | 60 |
| Molasses | 1 tbsp | 50 |
| Peanut butter | 1 tbsp | 95 |
| **VEGETABLES** | | |
| Baked beans | 1/2 cup | 150 |
| Broccoli (chopped) | 4 oz | 26 |
| Cabbage (cooked) | 1 cup | 30 |
| Carrots (cooked) | 1 cup | 45 |
| Cauliflower (cooked) | 1 cup | 25 |
| Celery (raw) | 8 in. stalk | 5 |
| Corn (canned) | 1 cup | 170 |
| Corn on the cob | 1 ear, 5 in. | 70 |
| Cucumber (raw) | 6 slices | 5 |

(continued)

## TABLE 9.1 *(continued)*

| FOOD DESCRIPTION | SERVING SIZE | APPROXIMATE CALORIES |
|---|---|---|
| **VEGETABLES** | | |
| Green bean and wax beans (cooked) | 1 cup | 30 |
| Lettuce | 3 large leaves | 10 |
| Onions (raw) | 1 medium | 40 |
| Peas (cooked) | 1 cup | 115 |
| Peppers, sweet green (raw) | 1 medium | 15 |
| Potatoes (baked) | 1 medium | 90 |
| Sweet potatoes (baked) | 1 medium | 155 |
| Radishes (raw) | 4 small | 5 |
| Spinach (cooked) | 1 cup | 40 |
| Squash, summer (cooked) | 1 cup | 30 |
| Squash, winter (cooked) | 1 cup | 130 |
| Tomato (raw) | 1 medium | 40 |
| Tomatoes, canned (cooked) | 1 cup | 50 |
| Tomato juice | 1 cup | 45 |
| **DESSERTS** | | |
| Apple pie (2 crusts) | 1/8 of 9 in. pie | 306 |
| Cashews | 1/4 cup | 196 |
| Chocolate chip cookies | one 2 in. | 70 |
| Chocolate fudge | 1 oz | 115 |
| Chocolate pudding | 1/2 cup | 193 |
| Cupcake with icing | 2 1/2 in. | 130 |
| Custard | 1 cup | 305 |
| Peanuts | 1/4 cup | 210 |
| Vanilla ice cream | 1/2 cup | 133 |
| **FISH** | | |
| Fish sticks (breaded) | 5 sticks of 4 oz each | 200 |
| Halibut (broiled) | One 4 oz | 205 |
| Lobster (meat only) | 4 oz | 100 |
| Perch (fried) | One 4 oz | 260 |
| Trout (fried) | 4 oz | 225 |
| Tuna (canned in oil) | 4 oz | 225 |
| Salmon (baked) | One 4 oz | 205 |
| **FRUITS AND JUICES** | | |
| Apple | 1 medium | 70 |
| Apple sauce | 1/2 cup | 115 |

*Basics for a Nutritious Diet* **233**

# TABLE 9.1 *(continued)*

| FOOD DESCRIPTION | SERVING SIZE | APPROXIMATE CALORIES |
|---|---|---|
| **FRUITS AND JUICES** | | |
| Banana | 1 medium | 100 |
| Grapefruit | 1/2 medium | 50 |
| Grapefruit juice (sweetened) | 4 fluid oz | 65 |
| Orange | 1 medium | 50 |
| Orange juice | 4 fluid oz | 55 |
| Rhubarb (cooked with sugar) | 1/2 cup | 193 |
| Watermelon | 4 × 8 inch wedge | 115 |
| **MISCELLANEOUS** | | |
| Catsup | 1 tbsp | 15 |
| Cole slaw (with mayonaise) | 1/2 cup | 255 |
| Mustard | 1 tbsp | 4 |
| Macaroni and cheese | 1 cup | 560 |
| Margarine (regular) | 1 tbsp | 100 |
| Marshmallow | 1 average size | 25 |
| Pickles, dill | 1 medium | 10 |
| Pickles, sweet | 1 medium | 20 |
| Pizza, with sauce & cheese | 1/4 of 12 in. pie | 575 |
| Popcorn, with oil & salt | 1 cup | 40 |
| Potato chips | 10 medium | 115 |
| Pretzels, thin twist | 1 twist | 25 |
| Relish | 1 tbsp | 20 |
| Spaghetti with meat sauce | 1 cup | 390 |
| Soybean oil | 1 tbsp | 125 |
| Tapioca | 1/2 cup | 280 |
| Tomato and lettuce salad (no dressing) | 1/2 cup | 60 |
| Tuna and celery salad (with mayonnaise) | 1/2 cup | 255 |
| **FAST FOOD STORES** | | |
| Arby's Roast Beef Sandwich | One regular | 429 |
| Burger King Whopper | One | 606 |
| Burger King Whaler | One | 744 |
| Colonel Sanders' Chicken | "3 piece special" | 660 |
| MacDonald's | Quarter pounder | 414 |
| | Quarter pounder with cheese | 521 |
| | Big Mac | 557 |

TABLE 9.1   *(continued)*

| FOOD DESCRIPTION | SERVING SIZE | APPROXIMATE CALORIES |
|---|---|---|
| FAST FOOD STORES | | |
| Pizza Hut | 1/2 of a 10 in. pizza | 440-490 |
| Arthur Treacher's Fish & Chips | 2 pieces of fish and 4 oz chips | 275 |
| Dairy Queen | Medium-sized cone | 339 |
| Dunkin Donuts | Plain with hole | 240 |
| | Yeast raised with filling | 250-260 |
| Baskin Robbins ice cream | One scoop with sugar cone | 180-230 |
| Most french fries | One package | 200 |
| Most milk shakes | Average size | 300 |

kilogram per minute, we get a total figure of 77.6 Calories/hour, or 1862 Calories/24 hours, a very close agreement.

The resting caloric need for a woman is calculated in the same manner, only with a 10-percent reduction. Thus, a 55-kilogram (121-lb) woman would utilize just under 1200 Calories a day (0.90 × 55 × 24).

To the basal metabolic value, you must add all caloric costs in excess of the resting expenditure of energy for the various activities that make up your day. The total represents your 24-hour caloric requirement. People's daily caloric expenditures vary considerably because of differences in their job requirements and recreational endeavors. It would be impractical to try to calculate your daily energy needs exactly every day. Table 9.2 provides an estimate of total daily caloric expenditures for men and women of different body weights and activity levels. Note that the lighter you are, the fewer Calories you require per day. Also, the less active you are, the fewer Calories you require.

If you wish to arrive at a close estimate of your caloric needs, follow the steps presented above for determining your basal metabolic rate. Then, using Table 9.2, select the figure that best describes your activity level. For instance, if you choose 60% multiply your resting rate (BMR) for 24 hours by 0.6. Add your result to the BMR. The total is an estimate of your total caloric expenditure for a 24-hour day. In order to maintain your present body weight, your daily caloric intake should equal the daily caloric expenditure you have calculated. If you want to lose, then reduce your daily intake of Calories below this level. The remainder of this chapter deals with

TABLE 9.2   ESTIMATED DAILY CALORIC EXPENDITURE FOR VARYING WEIGHTS AND ACTIVITY LEVELS* (CALORIES PER 24 HOURS)

| | MEN BODY WEIGHT | | | | WOMEN BODY WEIGHT | | | |
|---|---|---|---|---|---|---|---|---|
| | 60 kg (132 lb) | 70 kg (154 lb) | 80 kg (176 lb) | 90 kg (198 lb) | 50 kg (110 lb) | 55 kg (121 lb) | 60 kg (132 lb) | 65 kg (143 lb) |
| 40% Sedentary: physical activity limited to walking and sitting | 2030 | 2370 | 2710 | 3050 | 1520 | 1680 | 1830 | 1980 |
| 50% Semisedentary: engaged in activities which involve standing and walking | 2180 | 2540 | 2900 | 3270 | 1630 | 1790 | 1960 | 2120 |
| 60% Laborers: or limited physical exercise | 2320 | 2710 | 3100 | 3480 | 1740 | 1910 | 2090 | 2260 |
| 70% Heavy workers: regular participation in intramurals, sports, and other vigorous physical activities | 2470 | 2880 | 3290 | 3700 | 1850 | 2030 | 2220 | 2400 |
| 80% Engaged in intercollegiate sports or in a vigorous daily physical fitness program | 2610 | 3050 | 3480 | 3920 | 1960 | 2150 | 2350 | 2550 |

*Calculations have been based on a basal oxygen requirement of 3.5 milliliters of oxygen for each kilogram of body weight per minute and on a caloric equivalent of 4.8 Calories per liter of oxygen used. (Values listed have been rounded off to the nearest 10 Calories.)

regulating your diet and physical activity for either losing weight or maintaining your proper weight.

## OVERWEIGHT AND OBESITY

We all need the same nutrients, but in different amounts. Young people need greater quantities of food for body growth, upkeep, and energy. Men generally need more food than women; large people need more food than small people. However, when people overeat, that is, take in more Calories than their daily activities use up, they gain weight. Intake of food in excess of our daily needs leads to obesity, the state of being too fat.

Many people like to believe that some metabolic abnormality is the reason for their being overweight. Quite often this is not true. Medical research does not support the popular theory that endocrine malfunction is the reason for obesity. Instead, evidence is accumulating that our inactive sedentary way of life is the real culprit. We just don't burn off the Calories we eat each day. Thus the surplus energy is stored in the fat deposits of the body.

Recent research has indicated that human fat cells increase in number very rapidly in early life and, once formed, become fixed for life. Pediatricians are beginning to show a concern over this fact. A fat baby is not necessarily a healthy baby. Overfeeding tends to multiply the number of fat cells in the young child rapidly. It may even make it difficult for that child to control weight throughout his or her lifetime. To curb this potential for the

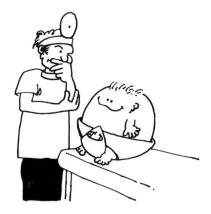

*A fat baby is not necessarily a healthy baby.*

unnecessary multiplying of fat cells, preventive steps must be taken at an early age through proper eating and exercise habits.

**Determining Relative Body Fat**

In determining your ideal weight, how fat you are is more important than how much you weigh. The standard age-height-weight tables are derived from measurements of a great number of people. Although these charts enable each person to make comparisons with the average man or woman, they are often inadequate guides to normal weight. Many athletes, low in body fat but very muscular, would be overweight according to these charts. Also, most of these age-height-weight charts allow small increments in body weight with increasing age, a practice that lacks justification.

Unmistakably, it is the proportion of fat tissue in your body, rather than your scale weight, that determines your proper weight. Fortunately,

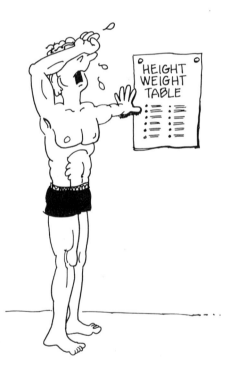

*Many people low in body fat but very muscular would be considered overweight according to height-weight tables.*

methods have been developed for measuring the relative leanness or fatness of the body. Skinfold calipers provide a simple means for estimating the percentage of body fat. These skinfold techniques correlate quite well with other, more complex methods for estimating body composition. (For example, one method is to weigh the body submersed in water; this technique determines the body's density and specific gravity. These measures are then used to estimate the proportions of lean body weight and body fat tissue. However, formulas based on skinfold measurements correlate quite well with this rather complex technique.)

Special calipers have been designed for measuring the skinfolds. Accuracy in their use, however, requires precise location of the site to be measured, firm pressure by the fingers in lifting the skinfold, and careful location of the point to which the calipers are applied. In Chapter 3, "Appraising Your Fitness," the use of calipers in determining relative body fat, along

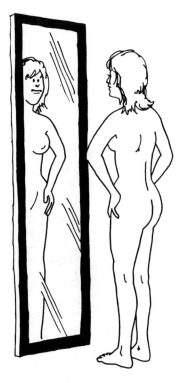

*Look at your naked body in front of a full-length mirror. If you look fat, you are fat!*

with a table of norms for men and women is discussed. A body fat value between 10 and 12 percent of the total body weight is considered ideal for adult men; by contrast, 18 to 20 percent body fat value for women generally signifies trim women. A value of over 25 percent in men, and over 30 percent in women, indicates obesity—too much fat.

If fat calipers are not available, an alternative is suggested. Look at your naked body in front of a full-length mirror. Observe your midsection, hip region, buttocks, and thighs. If you look fat, you are fat! Being able to pinch up about one inch of flabby fat between your fingers in some of these areas is a good indication of too much body fat. Remember, it is the proportion of fat tissue in the body's composition—rather than a reading on the bathroom scale—that determines if you are fat.

## THE ROLE OF EXERCISE IN WEIGHT CONTROL
The importance of regular exercise in weight control is well accepted today. Physical activity is the great variable in energy expenditure and can play a very important role in helping you control your body weight.

Few people view themselves as inactive, but in fact, studies have demonstrated that modern adults are increasingly less active than their counterparts in years gone by. Sedentary living is a sign of our times. Regular exercise and sound nutritional habits go hand-in-hand. Crash diets and crash exercise programs usually fail in the long run. As soon as the dieter resumes former eating habits, the excess weight is put back on. People

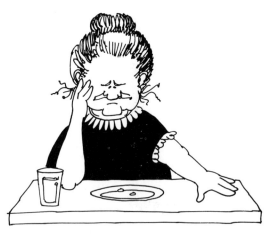

*For those who do not exercise regularly, the other alternative for weight control is sedentary living and life-long hunger.*

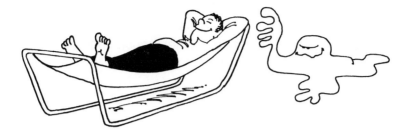

*Inactivity is the real culprit in "creeping obesity."*

who eat with discretion and exercise regularly, on the other hand, find weight control more feasible. The other alternative for weight control is sedentary living and lifelong hunger.

Inactivity has been shown over the years to be the real culprit in what is termed "creeping obesity." Studies comparing obese with nonobese subjects have demonstrated that the cause of fatness is usually an inactive life-style, not higher food consumption. However, despite the evidence for exercise as a means of weight control, several misunderstandings have tended to discredit exercise. One of these is the energy cost of various physical activities and their relative value for weight control.

**Energy Expenditure**

Recall that the heart rate during exercise is a direct reflection of the increased energy requirement. Accompanying the increased heart rate is an increase in the amount of blood pumped (cardiac output) and also an increase in oxygen uptake by muscle cells. This utilization of oxygen interrelates with the energy expenditure in the cells and is commonly expressed as Calories. The energy released during muscle contraction can be determined; it is known as the *energy expenditure* or, sometimes, as the *caloric cost.*

***Measurement of Energy Expenditure***

The caloric cost can be calculated if we can measure the amount of heat given off by the body. However, during exercise, this task has proven to be extremely difficult. During the late nineteenth century, a scientist related the heat loss from energy expenditure to the amount of oxygen consumed by the body. From this research a method, called *indirect calorimetry,* has been devised for measuring energy expenditure. Using it, we can calculate the number of Calories consumed by determining the amount of oxygen utilized. The validity of using rates of oxygen consumption as the basis for measuring energy expenditure has been firmly established.

### Oxygen Caloric Equivalency

One liter of oxygen consumed by the body during exercise is equivalent to approximately 5 Calories of expended energy. In other words, 1 Calorie is equivalent to 200 milliliters (0.2 liters) of oxygen consumed. For example, when walking at 3.5 mph, a person of average size uses about five Calories per minute, or 150 Calories in 30 minutes. Referring to the caloric values in Table 9.1 we see that a 12-ounce can of beer is also equivalent to 150 Calories or 30 minutes of walking. Understanding the relative energy values of food and physical activity will greatly assist you in carrying out a sound weight control program.

### Energy Cost of Activities

In recent years, much research has been devoted to establishing the energy costs of various sports and exercise activities. When estimating energy expenditure for any individual, we must consider the time spent in the activity, the rate of work, and body size. The more time you spend at an activity, the more energy you use. Larger people tend to require more energy than smaller people for the same task. Tables 9.3 and 9.4 dealing with energy cost express values in Calories per minute and in Calories per minute per kilogram of body weight. They will enable you to estimate your own caloric costs for selected activities.

These tables have been formulated from personal research and, in some cases, from research reported in professional journals. Activities that require 5 to 9 Cal/min (1.0 to 1.8 liters of oxygen) are classified as *moderate*. Activities requiring above 9 Cal/min are classified as *vigorous*. Table 9.3 presents Calorie-per-minute values for jogging and running for 120-, 150-, and 180-pound persons.

In addition, each jogging or running speed is expressed in terms of METS, another measure of caloric intensity. A MET refers to the rate of energy expended; one MET is equivalent to the energy needed at rest, or approximately 1.25 calories (about a quarter of a liter of oxygen). Classifying an activity at 7 METS, for instance, simply means that it requires seven times more energy than a state of rest. Seven METS would be at the high end of moderate exercise; it is equivalent to 8.8 Calories per minute, or a little more than 1.75 liters of oxygen uptake.

TABLE 9.3   ENERGY COST OF JOGGING AND RUNNING

| | CAL/MIN/KG | 120-LB PERSON (54 KG) | CAL/MIN 150-LB PERSON (68 KG) | 180-LB PERSON (81 KG) | METS RANGE |
|---|---|---|---|---|---|
| 10-min mile (6 mph) | 0.1471 | 7.9 | 10.0 | 11.9 | 6 to 10 |
| 8-min mile (7.5 mph) | 0.1856 | 10.0 | 12.6 | 15.0 | 8 to 12 |
| 7-min mile (8.6 mph) | 0.2118 | 11.4 | 14.4 | 17.2 | 9 to 14 |
| 6-min mile (10 mph) | 0.2350 | 12.7 | 16.0 | 19.0 | 10 to 15 |

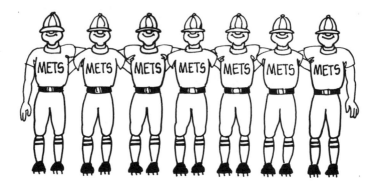

*Classifying an activity at 7 METS means that it requires 7 times more energy than a state of rest.*

Anything over 10 METS is considered very vigorous. Marathon runners, who probably represent the zenith of cardiorespiratory fitness, run for two to three hours at an intensity level of 12 to 15 METS or more.

For estimating your energy cost for jogging, first determine your kilogram body weight by multiplying your weight in pounds by 0.45 (1 pound equals 0.45 kilogram). Then select your preferred jogging speed. Multiply your kilogram weight by the value under the column headed Cal/min/kg. This will be the per-minute caloric cost for you.

For example, a 120-lb woman weighs 120 × 0.45 or 54.0 kg. Jogging at a 10-minute mile pace = 0.1471 × 54 = 7.9 Cal/min. This rate equals 237 Calories for 30 minutes of jogging. A value of 7.9 Cal/min would be classified at the high end of moderate. For a woman beginning a conditioning program, this level most likely represents an adequate intensity of exercise. However, as always, the key determining factor is the heart-rate response: it must be elevated to a level near 75% HR max to insure a training stimulus. (See Chapter 4 for determining your training heart rate.)

If we take a 170-pound man (76.5 kg) jogging at an 8-minute mile pace, he would require 14.2 Cal/minute. This is a greater caloric cost than for the example for a woman cited above. The reason for the higher cost is that he is jogging at a faster tempo and carrying more body mass. These factors require more energy. Nevertheless, the heart-rate response to this activity may or may not be 75% HR max—it all depends on his physical fitness. The better-conditioned you are, the greater the caloric expenditure you can muster in a given period of time. For example, contrast two men, both

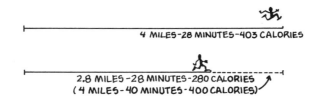

4 MILES-28 MINUTES-403 CALORIES

2.8 MILES -28 MINUTES-280 CALORIES
( 4 MILES-40 MINUTES-400 CALORIES)

weighing 68 kilograms. One can run for four miles in 28 minutes (a 7-minute mile pace) at a heart rate of 150 (an adequate training stimulus). The other can only run 2.8 miles during the same time period (28 minutes at a 10-minute pace) and at the same 150 heart rate. The first runner utilizes 403 Calories for his workout; the second man can utilize only 280 Calories during his workout. We can readily see that the man in better physical condition burns more Calories during his workout than the slower jogger does. This means more Calories expended, a bonus for weight control.

Now assume that the slower jogger goes four miles, in other words, the same total distance as the 28-minute jogger. He would then use another 120 Calories, which would give him a similar caloric expenditure, 400 Calories. However, his total workout time is 40 minutes rather than 28. Obviously, the jogger who can run the four miles in 28 minutes has a greater functional fitness capacity than the slow jogger. Nevertheless, *for burning Calories to control your weight, the most important factor is the distance you move, not the speed at which you move.*

Table 9.4 presents values for selected sports activities. The table is arranged in ascending order from the less intense activities (such as archery) to the most intense activity, running a 6-minute mile. Activities of below-moderate intensity, such as golf and archery, do not represent a suitable means for developing or maintaining physical fitness. In these sports the stress on the cardiorespiratory system is not great enough to produce a training effect. For weight control, however, activities such as golf can be beneficial. Although the cardiac and respiratory stimulus is very minimal, one does burn extra Calories. If we compare the 68-kilogram jogger who runs four miles in 28 minutes (a caloric cost of 403 Calories) with a golfer of the same weight, we find the golfer must play for a total of 106 minutes to burn the same 403 Calories (106 × 3.8). Put another way, the golfer has to play—exercise nearly four times as long for the same energy-cost benefits. And, as we have seen, the intensity of golf is not sufficient to produce a training effect on the heart and lungs. Low-intensity

TABLE 9.4   ENERGY COST OF SELECTED SPORTING ACTIVITIES

|  | CAL/MIN/KG | CAL/MIN* | METS* |
|---|---|---|---|
| Archery | | | |
| (American Round) | 0.0412 | 2.8 | 2.3 |
| Bowling (with three | | | |
| other bowlers) | 0.0471 | 3.2 | 2.7 |
| Golf (playing in | | | |
| a foursome) | 0.0559 | 3.8 | 3.2 |
| Walking (17-min mile on | | | |
| a grass surface) | 0.0794 | 5.4 | 4.5 |
| Cycling (6.4-min mile) | 0.0985 | 6.7 | 5.6 |
| Canoeing (15-min mile) | 0.1029 | 7.0 | 5.8 |
| Swimming (50-yd/min) | 0.1333 | 9.1 | 7.6 |
| Jogging (10-min mile) | 0.1471 | 10.0 | 8.0 |
| Cycling (5-min mile) | 0.1559 | 10.6 | 8.5 |
| Handball (singles) | 0.1603 | 10.9 | 9.1 |
| Rope skipping (80-turns/min) | 0.1655 | 11.3 | 9.5 |
| Jogging (8-min mile) | 0.1856 | 12.6 | 10.0 |
| Running (6-min mile) | 0.2350 | 16.0 | 12.8 |

*These are values for a 150-lb person (68 kg).

activities such as golf are not suitable for developing cardiorespiratory fitness.

## Common Misconceptions
Misconceptions about the relationship between exercise and weight control are quite common. Here are some of them.

### *Exercise and Appetite*
Often we hear that if you exercise more, you will eat more. Dr. Jean Mayer has systematically studied this theory. He has concluded that a daily exercise session does *not* bring about a corresponding increase in appetite and food intake. Appetite is a fairly good guide to the amount of food needed by active people, but it is not a reliable measure for inactive people. Therefore, it does not follow that if you are inactive you will eat less than if you were active. Mayer's observations suggest that there is a range of inactivity in which the level of food intake no longer correlates with a decrease in activity. In that range there is an imbalance between food intake and energy output, and fatness results. Mayer calls this the *sedentary range*.

Above this range of inactivity is the range of normal activity, where appetite and exercise are "attuned" to each other.

### Spot Reducing.

Health spas and weight reducing salons have often promoted spot reducing programs. Women, especially, are frequently encouraged to use localized exercise or mechanical vibrators and other gadgets to reduce the fatty stores in the areas of greatest fat deposition. However, the evidence available today does not support the theory that if you exercise a particular area of your body, you will reduce the excess fat from that region. Calisthenics, yoga, or "slimnastics" although beneficial to general muscle tone and flexibility, do not spot reduce.

However, several studies have indicated that regular exercise that is vigorous and continuous and that involves total body movement does reduce skinfold fat and girth measurements. The loss of fat, however, tends to be uniform all over the body, in proportion to the amount present at any given site. In contrast, exercises designed for exercising particular segments of the body do not appear to reduce fat in those areas. Calisthenics, combined with activities that vigorously stress the cardiorespiratory system, provide the best means for fat reduction.

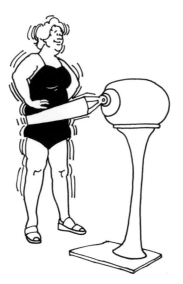

*Research evidence does not support the theory that you spot reduce an area of the body.*

### Weight Reduction by Sweating

Many people purposely overheat their bodies hoping for a quick loss of excess body weight. Exercising in hot, humid weather, or while wearing a rubber sweat suit, or even sitting in a steam room after exercise are common methods for prompting profuse sweating. Although one's reading on the scales may be temporarily a pound or two lower, this weight loss has nothing to do with body fat, and it will not be permanent. Basically, sweating procedures accomplish only one thing: a greater-than-normal loss of water from the body. This water loss, especially if excessive, can cause a serious problem. A rubber suit, or any unneeded extra clothing, does not allow the heat produced during exercise to escape from the body. Also, a steam room or a hot humid environment diminishes the body's capacity to dispel heat normally. Evaporation of sweat is the major means for heat dissipation at the surface of the skin during vigorous exercise. When one wears a rubber suit, the heat and sweat given off between the suit and the skin are trapped, causing body temperature to become greater than normal. Body

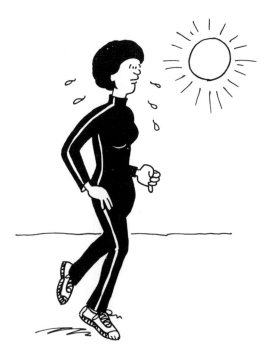

*Dehydration is useless for weight control and can be dangerous.*

heat rises, but the trapped sweat is unable to evaporate. Eventually, body heat is raised beyond its normal range. Failure of the heat produced by the exercising muscles to be eliminated properly imposes an added burden on the heat-regulating mechanisms. This leads to a loss of too much body water and, in turn, a decrease in blood volume, a severe rise in body temperature, and possible circulatory collapse. These events, if severe enough, can produce heat stroke and death.

The key point here is that dehydration (removal of body water) is useless for weight control and can be dangerous. Even if you are careful to limit overeating, you will restore the depleted body water in a few hours when you eat and drink. Water does not contain calories, and excess body weight (fat) is only lost by burning calories, not by losing water. Therefore these weight-reducing practices are not only useless, they are also dangerous. Tampering with the heat balance of the body can be risky. But sweating itself is not a hazard, it is a necessary mechanism for maintaining heat balance during physical activity.

## A PLAN FOR LOSING WEIGHT

Exercise has often been scoffed at as a means of reducing or controlling weight. The accepted figure for melting off a pound of fat is 3500 Calories. Even if you exercised very vigorously for 30 minutes, you would be hard pressed to burn 500 Calories. Thus it would take seven days to lose a pound of fat by exercise alone (7 × 500). However, if you take a long-range view of the situation and exercise at a more reasonable caloric level of 300 Calories (one you can endure) for four days a week, you would be spending an extra 1200 Calories a week. Thus, if you maintained your food intake at a constant level and exercised for four days a week you would lose about 15 pounds a year.

If you combine vigorous exercise with a reduced diet, you have a very effective means for shedding excess poundage. Again, if you exercise four days a week at 300 Calories per session, but also reduce your daily food intake by 400 Calories you have a 4000-Calorie deficit per week. This program theoretically would bring about a weight loss of approximately one pound of fat a week. For many people anxious to lose weight this seems to be too slow a process. However, experience has demonstrated that body weight lost gradually and systematically has a greater tendency to stay off. Figure 9.1 illustrates some of the possible relationships between daily caloric intake and daily caloric expenditure.

Inactivity is the dominant feature in the caloric balance of most over-

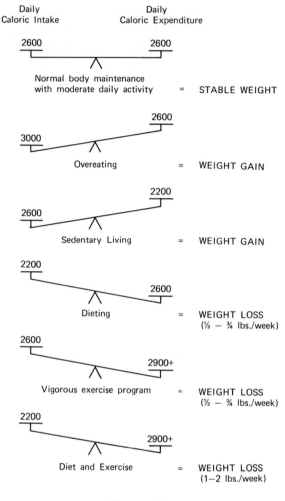

| Daily Caloric Intake | Daily Caloric Expenditure | | |
|---|---|---|---|
| 2600 | 2600 | | |
| Normal body maintenance with moderate daily activity | | = | STABLE WEIGHT |
| 3000 | 2600 | = | WEIGHT GAIN |
| Overeating | | | |
| 2600 | 2200 | = | WEIGHT GAIN |
| Sedentary Living | | | |
| 2200 | 2600 | = | WEIGHT LOSS (½ — ¾ lbs./week) |
| Dieting | | | |
| 2600 | 2900+ | = | WEIGHT LOSS (½ — ¾ lbs./week) |
| Vigorous exercise program | | | |
| 2200 | 2900+ | = | WEIGHT LOSS (1—2 lbs./week) |
| Diet and Exercise | | | |

*Figure 9.1*

weight people. The ability to sit all day without getting fat has not been bred into the human being.

### Approximating Your Desired Weight

Once you have an estimate of your percentage of body fat (by the skinfold method) you can estimate your desired weight. Based on the formulas we recommend, body fat values of 18 percent for women and 12 percent for men appear to represent reasonable targets for young adults.

Let's take an example. A young man weighs 86 kg (189 lb), and his percentage of body fat is estimated at 23%. This figures to 19.8 kg of body fat (0.23 × 86) and 66.2 kg of lean body weight (86 − 19.8). To calculate his body weight at 12 percent fat, we simply divide the lean body weight by 0.88. We get a value of 75 kg, or 165 pounds, as his ideal body weight. By using an 18 percent standard for women, we divide the lean body weight (fatfree weight) by 0.82. These figures are only estimates; however, for many years this method has proved to be very worthwhile for setting goals for weight reduction. (See Chapter 3, "Appraising Your Fitness," for a more detailed method of determining relative fat and your desired weight.)

## LIFETIME CONCEPT OF WEIGHT CONTROL

Food has always been a center of our life. Eating, although a necessity, can also be viewed as a recreation—something we do in leisure time for pleasure. We snack in front of the TV set or at an athletic event; we go out to eat at our favorite restaurants. Preparation of hearty and tasty meals is a way of showing affection for others; holiday feasts, cocktail parties, and backyard barbecues are part of one's social routine. Business transactions are frequently conducted over food and drink. The result of all this enjoyable abandon can be excess poundage or even outright obesity.

We live in a society that has become increasingly inactive with the advancement of technology. Today, sedentary living is being encouraged with the continued development of automated work-savers and the promotion of passive amusements and recreation. With the consumption of a poor but plentiful diet, complicated by the tensions of everyday living characteristic of modern times, a very dismal picture unveils for maintaining an optimal level of health and appearance. Keep in mind that the body was made to be active and it thrives on movement and vigorous activity. An active life-style should be programmed into your daily living plan to counter the effects of technological advances. You need to blend proper eating habits with vigorous exercise to develop and maintain a healthy functioning body.

Obesity and inactivity have been correlated with coronary heart disease, high blood pressure, diabetes, and other degenerative disorders. But obesity and fatness are practically unknown among vigorous, active people. Athletes, joggers, and active sportsmen seldom have excess body fat. The purpose of this chapter has been to provide a sound basis for understanding nutrition and weight control. Exercise can be the key mediator in this process. A sound, nutritious diet combined with regular vigorous exercise is the best strategy for a lifetime of successful weight control. The goal is not merely to lose fat but to keep it off, or better still, never to put it on. Therefore, now is the time to establish sound nutritional and exercise habits. Don't wait until your health is in peril.

## KEY WORDS

AMINO ACIDS: The end product of the breakdown of protein.

BASAL METABOLIC RATE (BMR): The minimal rate of energy required to maintain the life processes of the body during a resting state following at least twelve hours of not eating.

BLOOD SUGAR: The glucose concentration in the blood. This term should not be confused with refined sugar. See SUGAR.

CALORIE: A unit of measure for the rate of heat or energy production in the body.

CARBOHYDRATES: A food substance that is the primary energy food for vigorous muscular activity. Includes various sugars and starches and is found in the body in the form of glucose and glycogen.

FAT: A food substance used as a source of energy in the body and is capable of being stored.

FATTY ACID: The end product of the breakdown of fats.

GLUCOSE: The end product of carbohydrate transported in the blood (blood sugar) and metabolized in the cell.

GLYCOGEN: The form in which carbohydrates are stored in the muscles and liver.

GRAM: A unit of mass and weight in the metric system. An ounce equals 28.3 grams, whereas 1000 grams equals one kilogram or 2.2 pounds.

KILOGRAM: Metric measure of weight; 2.2 pounds equals one kilogram or 1000 grams.

LEAN BODY WEIGHT: The body weight minus the percent of body weight that is stored fat.

MET: Represents the rate of energy expended at rest and used to rate activities in multiples above rest.

MINERALS: A group of 22 metallic elements that are vital to proper cell functioning; for example, minerals are part of enzymes, hormones, and vitamins.

NUTRIENT: The basic substances of the body that are provided by the eating of foods.

NUTRITION: The study of food and how the body uses it.

OBESITY: An excessive amount of body fat or the state of being too fat.

OXYGEN UPTAKE: Indicates the amount of energy the body uses; can be easily converted to Calories.

PROTEIN: A food substance that provides the basic structural properties of the cells and is also the source for enzymes and hormones in the body.

RELATIVE BODY FAT: The proportion of fat tissue in your body, often expressed as a percentage of body weight.

SATURATED FATS: A food source found in meat, milk, cheese, and butter. This type of fat does not melt at room temperature.

SUGAR: A term often misused; in this book it refers to refined sugar or table sugar; the scientific name for sugar is sucrose. See BLOOD SUGAR.

UNSATURATED FATS: A liquid type of fat found in peanut oil and olive oil.

VITAMINS: Organic substances that perform vital functions within the cells.

# SUPPLEMENTARY READINGS

Brody, Jane, "How I lost 35 pounds and kept them off," *Family Circle.* **91:**104, April 24, 1978.

Buskirk, Elsworth and Emily Haymes, "Nutritional Requirements for Women in Sport," *Women and Sport: A National Research Conference.* Dorothy V. Harris, ed., Pennsylvania State University, 1972, pages 339–374.

Higdon, Hal (ed.), *The Complete Diet Guide For Runners and Other Athletes.* Mountain View, California: World Publications, 1978.

Katch, Frank I. and William D. McArdle, *Nutrition, Weight Control, and Exercise.* Boston: Houghton Mifflin, 1977.

Mayer, Jean, *A Diet for Living.* New York: Pocket Books, 1977.

Mayer, Jean, *Overweight: Causes, Cost and Control.* Englewood Cliffs, New Jersey: Prentice-Hall, 1968.

Mayer, Jean, "Sugar: Taking the Bitter with the Sweet," *Family Health.* **10:**26–27, February, 1978.

Oscai, Larry, "The Role of Exercise in Weight Control," *Exercise and Sports Sciences Reviews,* Jack H. Wilmore, ed. New York: Academic Press, 1973.

"The Perils of Eating, American Style," *Time.* **100:**68–76, December 18, 1972.

Vantallie, Theodore, "Trouble Losing Weight?" *U.S. News & World Report.* **77:**56–58, July 22, 1974.

# chapter ten

Although there appears to be a decline in recent years in the American heart mortality rate, the United States still leads the world in deaths due to heart disease. Equally distressing is the fact that the leading cause of death in the 35 to 44 age bracket is still coronary heart disease. Even though the death rates of men are much higher than those for women, American women lead those of all other countries in heart disease rates.

As you read this chapter give thought to the following statements:

• Heart disease occurs when the coronary arteries (the blood vessels that supply the heart muscle with nutrients and oxygen) are impaired by a build-up of cholesterol and associated fatty substances on the inner portion of the artery wall. Such accumulations (often referred to as atherosclerosis) tend to limit the blood flow to the heart muscle and such blockage, if severe enough, can lead to heart attack.

• Medical research has identified certain "risk factors" associated with an increased incidence of atherosclerosis. Such factors as high blood pressure, smoking, and a high level of fats in the blood are highly related to the occurrence of heart disease. Many other variables such as obesity, lack of exercise, everyday tensions, and diabetes have also been correlated with atherosclerosis.

• One's age, sex, and heredity are risk factors that cannot be readily controlled or remedied. However, proper diet and exercise offer some protection against the early appearance of heart disease.

• Vigorous exercise, properly adhered to on a regular basis, appears to have much potential for adding more "life to your years" and possibly more "years to your life."

# activity and heart disease

Coronary heart disease is the leading cause of death in the United States today. Over one million heart attacks occur each year, resulting in more than 650,000 deaths. The American heart mortality rate is the highest in the world. According to estimates by the American Heart Association, over 53 percent of all American deaths in 1978 were caused by disease of the cardiovascular system (the heart and blood vessels). Despite significant advances in the recognition and treatment of heart disease, the unfortunate fact is that heart deaths have only slightly declined in recent years. Equally discouraging is the statistic that coronary heart disease is the leading cause of death among males in the 35 to 44 age bracket. In fact, of all coronary heart disease deaths in 1975, more than a third were men under age 65. The mortality rates for men are several times higher than those for women. Nevertheless, American women lead those of all other countries in heart disease death rates.

Some experts call heart disease the "disease of prosperity"; others label it the "abuse of our prosperity." The accomplishments of technology, automation, and science have raised our living standards. However, the resultant soft living has made us vulnerable targets for heart disease. Research is showing that regular exercise can help counteract the effects of our life-style.

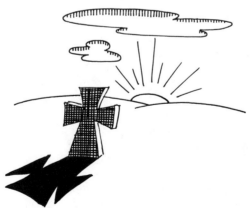

*Coronary heart disease is the leading cause of death in the United States today.*

## ATHEROSCLEROSIS

The heart is a sturdy, tough muscle; it contracts 100,000 times a day with enough force to pump blood through 60,000 miles of blood vessels. The blood pumped through the heart, however, does not nourish the heart itself. Instead, the heart muscle is supplied with blood through its own system, the coronary arteries.

Coronary heart disease occurs when these arteries are impaired by a buildup of cholesterol and associated fatty substances on the inner portion of the artery wall. These deposits cause a thickening of the inner walls and a serious narrowing of the blood vessels, a condition called atherosclerosis. In later stages these deposits cause the arteries to lose their pliability which leads to a hardening of the vessels, termed arteriosclerosis. When such accumulations occur in the coronary arteries, they limit the blood flow to the heart muscle. When the blockage becomes severe, the heart can suffer a myocardial infarction, the death of part of the heart muscle. This malfunction may seem sudden, but it has actually been building up to this crisis for years.

The best evidence of the early and gradual accumulation of fatty deposits in the body's arteries is a much-quoted study of 300 United States soldiers killed in the Korean War. The subjects averaged only 22 years of age, but 77 percent of them showed signs of diseases of the coronary arteries, varying from a slight thickening of the artery linings to complete occlusion (blockage) of one or more main artery branches. A substantial proportion of these young Americans had impaired circulation long before any symptoms would have appeared. Interestingly, comparable studies of

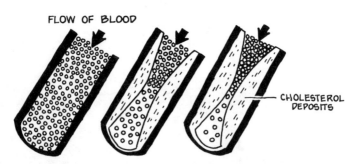

FLOW OF BLOOD

CHOLESTEROL DEPOSITS

*Coronary heart disease occurs when the coronary arteries are impaired by the buildup of cholesterol and associated fatty substances on the inner portion of the artery wall.*

Korean soldiers killed alongside the Americans revealed no evidence of similar coronary damage. Studies in other countries (such as autopsies of accident victims) showed again that early atherosclerosis is more common in young American men than it is elsewhere in the world.

From this evidence we must realize that coronary heart disease is not simply a disease of the elderly. Instead, this deadly buildup of fatty substances in the arteries begins at an early age. Some pediatricians feel that preventive measures should begin in childhood and perhaps even in infancy. Heart disease doesn't just happen overnight; it may well begin in childhood and lead to a heart attack in the prime of life.

## CORONARY RISK FACTORS

Recently medical attention has been directed at the prevention of coronary heart disease. Extensive research has identified certain so-called "risk factors" that are associated with an increased incidence of atherosclerosis. The greater the number of these coronary risk factors one has, the greater one's chance for heart disease, and perhaps premature death. High blood pressure (hypertension), high levels of fats (cholesterol and triglycerides) in the blood, diabetes, obesity, cigarette smoking, emotional behavior, and inactivity all have been linked to coronary heart disease. Other factors involve one's age, sex, race, and heredity. The latter are pre-determined and cannot be readily controlled or remedied. However, we can do something about diet, body fatness, smoking, and exercise.

### Age, Sex, Race, and Genetic Factors

The incidence of atherosclerosis and coronary heart disease increases with age. The death rate among American white males is about 10 in 100,000 at ages 25 to 34; at ages 55 to 64 it increases to almost 1000 in 100,000. The American Heart Association estimated that in 1975, one-fourth of all persons killed by cardiovascular diseases were under age 65.

At ages 35 to 44, the death rate of white males from coronary heart disease is 6.1 times that of women. However, after menopause, the incidence of the disease for women nearly approaches the level of men of comparable age. The women's diminished hormonal production after menopause is believed to account for this increased coronary disease rate.

Black people have a higher death rate from coronary heart disease than white people do. Surprisingly, the black woman is stricken at an earlier age than the white man or woman, and even earlier than black men. The reason for this circumstance is not clear.

A hereditary element is linked with coronary disease. Heart attacks, especially those that strike at an early age, appear to run in families. However, the specific genetic defects remain unknown. There is some speculation that this relationship is environmental rather than genetic. For example, fat parents usually have fat children; tense parents often create tense children; and poor dietary habits and inactive life-styles are often family-influenced. The exact nature of the role of heredity in coronary heart disease is very complex, especially when we consider the other conditions that frequently precede coronary heart disease, such as diabetes, hypertension, and elevated serum cholesterol. In some instances, these factors can be inherited; however, they are also outcomes of one's living style.

## Hypertension

If you have ever had a physical examination, most likely your blood pressure has been checked. An inflatable cuff is wrapped on your arm, and air is pumped into the cuff. Indirectly this procedure measures the amount of pressure maintained in your arteries. The pumping ability of your heart and the resiliency of your arteries influence the measurement. The pressure is recorded in two numbers. The high number, called systolic pressure, is your blood pressure at the moment blood is ejected from the heart. The lower number, the diastolic pressure, is your blood pressure between beats when the heart is relaxed and resting. Under relaxed conditions the pressure rises from a diastolic level of 80 mm Hg (millimeters of mercury) to a systolic level of 120 mm Hg. The pressure is capable of going up and down within a limited range (as during exercise), but when it starts high and stays high during rest, it is called hypertension. High blood pressure, which usually means any pressures above 140/90, is largely unexplained. However, it has been strongly linked to heart disease. Control of hypertension has improved recently with the development of effective drugs. Exercise also helps to reduce the arterial pressure in some people. Unfortunately, more than half of the 24 million Americans who are hypertensive don't know it. And many who are aware of it are not getting suitable treatment. A man with a systolic blood pressure of over 150 mm Hg has more than twice the risk of heart attack than men with systolic pressure under 120. Do you know what your own blood pressure is?

## Cholesterol and Triglycerides

The relationship between high blood cholesterol levels and heart disease has provoked much controversy for more than a decade. Cholesterol is produced in the liver; it is essential for cell structure and for the formation of various hormones, the sex hormones included. However, cholesterol and another fatty substance called triglycerides also make up the atherosclerotic deposits on the inner lining of the arteries. Medical researchers believe that cholesterol floating in the blood is the source of the continual accumulation. A diet high in saturated fat increases cholesterol concentrations in the blood.

The level of cholesterol in the blood can be measured. Any value above 250 mg per 100 ml of blood is considered dangerous. According to the American Heart Association, a man with a value of 250 or more mg per 100 ml, for instance, has about three times the risk of heart attack or stroke as a man with a cholesterol level below 200. Diets high in animal fat and high cholesterol foods, and an inactive life-style have both been identified as factors correlated with high cholesterol levels. Recent evidence has shown the worth of substituting some of the saturated fats in the diet with polyunsaturated fats derived from vegetable sources, such as safflower oil. This adjustment in diet has tended to lower cholesterol values in some people. There is some evidence of reductions in cholesterol level as the result of physical fitness programs, but the role of exercise as a controlling agent for cholesterol is still not generally accepted.

Triglycerides are "true" fat particles and represent 95 percent of the total fats stored in the body. In recent years the measurement of triglycerides in the blood has been carried out to provide an index of the number of fatty particles floating around in the blood stream. When excessive amounts of carbohydrates (sugar and starches) are eaten and they are not used for energy, the excess is turned into fats (triglycerides). Triglycerides provide the main means for fat to be transported in the blood. When fat is not used for immediate energy, the excess is stored within fat cells that are situated throughout the body (such as your abdomen, thighs, arms, chin, etc.). These fats also appear to be associated with atherosclerosis and, like cholesterol, can be lowered by weight loss, diet restrictions, and exercise. In fact, recent research has shown dramatic drops of triglyceride levels with endurance exercise. A high carbohydrate diet tends to be reflected in high triglyceride levels. Also, daily consumption of cocktails (alcohol) may be a reason for elevated triglycerides. The normal range of triglycerides is 10 to 150 mg%. Many active people fall well below the 100 mg% value.

Although it is important to keep your levels of cholesterol and triglycerides down, new findings from several heart disease studies suggest a more involved analysis of blood lipids. The medical thinking now is that it may be more important to know how cholesterol is carried in the bloodstream rather than just knowing the total amount present. Cholesterol is carried in the bloodstream by certain proteins. Because these proteins are carrying a lipid they are called lipoproteins. Three types of lipoprotein are especially important to heart disease: high density lipoprotein (HDL), low density lipoprotein (LDL), and very low density lipoprotein (VLDL). The VLDLs are responsible for transporting triglycerides (which result from eating excess carbohydrates and calories) from the liver to the fat cells for storage throughout the body. The LDLs carry cholesterol from the liver to the cells of various tissues where it is used to make cell membranes and certain hormones. For years medicine has known that the cholesterol being deposited in the arteries (atherosclerosis) is the cholesterol attached to the LDL. In contrast, the HDL had as its major function to clear unneeded cholesterol from the tissues and return it to the liver to be excreted. Although not clearly established, HDLs are thought to prevent cholesterol from depositing on the inner walls of the arteries, thus "thwarting" the process of atherosclerosis. In other words, evidence is accumulating that people who have high levels of HDL-cholesterol in their blood tend to be relatively free of heart disease whereas those with high LDL levels are more likely to suffer heart attacks. In a recent publication on the Framingham heart study it was emphasized that high-density-lipoprotein cholesterol is the most powerful single lipid predictor of coronary artery disease. In addition, recent reports indicate that middle-aged runners tend to have increased and higher levels of HDL when compared with nonactive people. There also appears to be less LDL among these runners. Although it may be too early to say, these preliminary studies suggest a strong case for vigorous exercise as a preventive measure for coronary heart disease.

A survey was reported in 1976 concerning the dietary habits, blood lipid levels, and degree of fatness for over 3000 people in a Michigan community. The study inferred that the degree of fatness of an individual was a more obvious determinant of high blood fats than the nutritional composition of the diet. The authors cautioned that these results do not mean that diet and lipid levels are unrelated. It was suggested that attainment and maintenance of desirable body weight is a worthy goal for prevention and control of hyperlipidemia (high blood fats) in the general population. With this in mind and the recent research suggesting that endurance activity (such as running) increases the high density lipoproteins in the blood and reduces the low density lipoproteins, a validity is evident for the beneficial effects of exercise as a preventive measure to heart disease.

## Diabetes

Quite often <u>diabetes</u> is a hereditary disease, especially when it appears at an early age. People with diabetes have a high incidence of atherosclerosis. In diabetics the severity of coronary heart disease is greater, the death rate is higher, and there is an increased incidence of premature heart attack. Female diabetics have a coronary death rate that is 6.4 times that of a nondiabetic woman. Diabetes, in other words, negates the protection from coronary heart disease that young women normally enjoy. The actual connection between diabetes and heart disease is not known. One theory suggests that diabetes results in increased fat deposits in the arteries. Again, diet management is crucial. If your family has a history of diabetes mellitus, you should have a glucose tolerance test.

Recent findings are suggesting that *regular* vigorous physical activity for the diabetic is beneficial because it helps to clear sugars and fats from the blood. In other words, exercise lowers the blood glucose without the use of <u>insulin</u>. Dr. David Costill, Director of the Human Performance Laboratory at Ball State University, has been studying the responses of diabetics to exercise. He and his associates have observed that a diabetic who exercises for 30 or more minutes daily may show as much as 30 to 40 percent reduction in the need for insulin.

## Obesity

Obesity (excessive fat) is one disease clearly evident in our society. Ten to 20 percent of children are overweight and 35 to 50 percent of all middle-aged Americans are overweight. The high relationship of obesity with high blood pressure and other circulatory diseases clearly implicates the seriousness of being overfat.

Health problems of an obese person may not be caused by the overweight condition but may be linked with a disorder such as heart disease. For example, some individuals with high blood pressure are obese. A substantial weight loss may lower their blood pressure. Also, with the consumption of too much food, especially saturated fats, the fat levels in the blood tend to be high. A high concentration of fats in the blood correlates with the presence of atherosclerosis and increases the risk of a coronary heart attack.

During physical work, obesity imposes an increased load on the heart and it limits exercise tolerance. Obesity is a health hazard. Although it may not cause heart disease, it does create an extra risk for otherwise healthy people. This alone justifies weight reduction as a sound health measure for

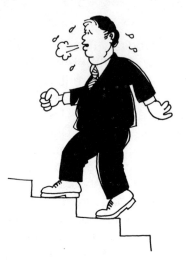

*Obesity imposes an increased load on the heart during physical work.*

possible prevention of heart disease or other related disorders. In Chapter 9 suggestions are given for combining a sound nutritious diet with regular vigorous exercise for a lifetime of successful weight control.

### Smoking

It is generally agreed that cigarette smoking is harmful to health. No person has ever benefited from smoking. That seems to be putting it mildly when we survey the documented evidence against smoking. Its connection with pulmonary emphysema and lung cancer as well as with heart attacks certainly do not make smoking a very healthy recreation. However, the exact

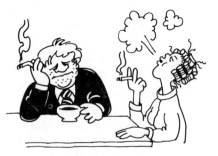

*No person has ever benefited from smoking.*

role that smoking plays in the development of heart attacks has not been established. The current belief is that smoking doesn't cause atherosclerosis, but it may more readily trigger a heart attack in a person whose vessels are already clogged. The American Heart Association states that a person smoking more than one pack a day has nearly twice the risk of heart attack of the nonsmoker.

## Type A Behavior
Quite recently much consideration has been given to the possible relationship of one's daily behavior pattern to heart disease. Few medical researchers in the past have bothered to focus on one's mental and emotional processes and their influence on the health of the heart. Drs. Friedman and Rosenman in their book, *Type A Behavior and Your Heart,* believe that the major cause of coronary heart disease is a complex of emotional reactions to environmental and societal agents that force us to live and work continuously faster. It is their strong belief that these chronic emotional upsets lead to excessive biochemical changes in the body that are detrimental to the heart. Such events lead to increased cholesterol levels and other abnormal changes in the body. A sense of "time urgency" (a chronic incessant struggle to achieve more and more in less and less time) and a demonstration of "free floating" hostility (a tendency to compete aggressively with others) are the main destructive Type A forces that appear to be characteristic of many individuals suffering from coronary disease. A research study disclosed that 70 percent of a group of coronary-stricken men exhibited characteristics of "excessive competitive drive and an urgency for meeting deadlines." Thus they strongly recom-

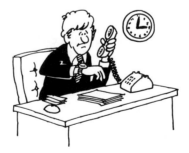

*Excessive competitive drive and an urgency for meeting deadlines are Type A characteristics.*

mend that alteration of Type A behavior is the chief factor for preventing a heart attack.

From our own experiences in conducting exercise programs, we strongly believe that participation in vigorous rhythmical exercise, as recommended throughout this book, has great potential for offsetting some of the tensions and mental stresses characteristic of Type A behavior. Much has been written about the psychological benefits of exercise, specifically running. James Fixx in his best seller *The Complete Book of Running* devotes a complete chapter to "What happens to your mind." Enhanced mental energy, increased concentration, greater confidence, and an improved ability to relax are some of the many attributes mentioned by Fixx that are associated with running. A San Diego Psychiatrist, Dr. Thaddeus Kostrubala, in his book, *The Joy of Running,* also promotes the psychological and mental benefits of running.

An increasing number of people are finding that they can enjoy a more positive mental well-being if they get regular physical activity. Reports of more adequate sleep and feelings of better health are quite common among "active" people. Although most of the evidence concerning Type A behavior is empirical, it still warrants consideration, along with the other risk factors, as something we all should confront in seeking a life of health and well-being.

## Inactivity

The study of the relationship between physical inactivity and heart disease has produced conflicting data. Sedentary living is recognized as a risk factor, but of lesser influence when compared with the well-known risk factors: high levels of blood fat, high blood pressure, and smoking.

Regular, vigorous exercise is a part of good health and well-being. There is little dispute that rhythmic exercise such as jogging, cycling, and swimming can measurably improve the efficiency of the heart and circulation. In fact, evidence is beginning to suggest that it can be a very effective measure in preventing premature heart disease.

By now the multitude of factors that cause coronary heart disease should be quite clear. We are limited by what we can do about some of these factors, such as heredity, sex, race, and age. Nevertheless, we can do something about the other risk factors (diet, obesity, smoking, and inactivity). Assuming coronary risk factors are associated directly with the chances of being afflicted with coronary heart disease and that physical activity can influence some of the risk factors, then exercise aimed at improving cardiorespiratory fitness may be the key to preventing or reducing mortality from coronary heart disease.

## WHAT IS YOUR RISK?

What are your chances of suffering a heart attack? Here is a simple test, developed by the Michigan Heart Association in 1969 (see illustration). This

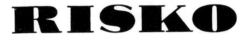

The purpose of this game is to give you an estimate of your chances of suffering heart attack.

The game is played by making squares which — from left to right — represent an increase in your RISK FACTORS. These are medical conditions and habits associated with an increased danger of heart attack. Not all risk factors are measurable enough to be included in this game; see back of sheet for other RISK FACTORS.

RULES:

Study each RISK FACTOR AND its row. Find the box applicable to you and circle the large number in it. For example, if you are 37, circle the number in the box labeled 31--40.

After checking out all the rows, add the circled numbers. This total — your score — is an estimate of your risk.

IF YOU SCORE:

6--11 — Risk well below average

12--17 — Risk below average

18--24 — Risk generally average

25--31 — Risk moderate

32--40 — Risk at a dangerous level

41--62 — Danger urgent. See your doctor now.

HEREDITY:

Count parents, grand--parents, brothers, and sisters who have had heart attack and/or stroke.

TOBACCO SMOKING:

If you inhale deeply and smoke a cigarette way down, add one to your classification. Do NOT subtract because you think you do not inhale or smoke only a half inch on a cigarette.

EXERCISE:

Lower your score one point if you exercise regularly and frequently.

CHOLESTEROL OR SATURATED FAT INTAKE LEVEL:

A cholesterol blood level is best. If you can't get one from your doctor, then estimate honestly the percentage of solid fats you eat. These are usually of animal origin — lard, cream, butter, and beef and lamb fat. If you eat much of this, your cholesterol level probably will be high. The U.S. average, 40%, is too high for good health.

BLOOD PRESSURE:

If you have no recent reading but have passed an insurance or industrial examination chances are you are 140 or less.

SEX:

This line takes into account the fact that men have from 6 to 10 times more heart attacks than women of child bearing age.

*RISKO is reprinted courtesy of Michigan heart Association and © Michigan heart Association.*

| | | | | | | |
|---|---|---|---|---|---|---|
| **AGE** | **1**<br>10 to 20 | **2**<br>21 to 30 | **3**<br>31 to 40 | **4**<br>41 to 50 | **6**<br>51 to 60 | **8**<br>61 to 70<br>and over |
| **HEREDITY** | **1**<br>No known history of heart disease | **2**<br>1 relative with cardiovascular disease<br>Over 60 | **3**<br>2 relatives with cardiovascular disease<br>Over 60 | **4**<br>1 relative with cardiovascular disease<br>Under 60 | **6**<br>2 relatives with cardiovascular disease<br>Under 60 | **7**<br>3 relatives with cardiovascular disease<br>Under 60 |
| **WEIGHT** | **0**<br>More than 5 lbs. below standard weight | **1**<br>−5 to +5 lbs. standard weight | **2**<br>6–20 lbs. over weight | **3**<br>21–35 lbs. over weight | **5**<br>36–50 lbs. over weight | **7**<br>51–65 lbs. over weight |
| **TOBACCO SMOKING** | **0**<br>Non-user | **1**<br>Cigar and/or pipe | **2**<br>10 cigarettes or less a day | **4**<br>20 cigarettes a day | **6**<br>30 cigarettes a day | **10**<br>40 cigarettes a day or more |
| **EXERCISE** | **1**<br>Intensive occupational and recreational exertion | **2**<br>Moderate occupational and recreational exertion | **3**<br>Sedentary work and intense recreational exertion | **5**<br>Sedentary occupational and moderate recreational exertion | **6**<br>Sedentary work and light recreational exertion | **8**<br>Complete lack of all exercise |
| **CHOLES-TEROL OR FAT % IN DIET** | **1**<br>Cholesterol below 180 mg. %<br>Diet contains no animal or solid fats | **2**<br>Cholesterol 181–205 mg. %<br>Diet contains 10% animal or solid fats | **3**<br>Cholesterol 206–230 mg. %<br>Diet contains 20% animal or solid fats | **4**<br>Cholesterol 231–255 mg. %<br>Diet contains 30% animal or solid fats | **5**<br>Cholesterol 256–280 mg. %<br>Diet contains 40% animal or solid fats | **7**<br>Cholesterol 281–300 mg. %<br>Diet contains 50% animal or solid fats |
| **BLOOD PRESSURE** | **1**<br>100 upper reading | **2**<br>120 upper reading | **3**<br>140 upper reading | **4**<br>160 upper reading | **6**<br>180 upper reading | **8**<br>200 or over upper reading |
| **SEX** | **1**<br>Female under 40 | **2**<br>Female 40–50 | **3**<br>Female over 50 | **5**<br>Male | **6**<br>Stock male | **7**<br>Bald stocky male |

test, set up as a game, assesses the main risk factors associated with heart attacks. The game, called *Risko,* involves assigning yourself the appropriate numerical value in each of the risk categories on the chart. You then add up the numbers. The sum represents your overall risk. If you score a total above 24, it is recommended that you seek medical consultation. Although Risko is no substitute for a medical examination, it does provide immediate information about your chances of suffering a heart attack.

## CARDIAC REHABILITATION
The role of physical exercise has been shown to be a key tool for the rehabilitation of cardiac patients. Exercise helps restore not only the physical functions of the body but also enhances psychological, social, and spiritual qualities. The safety of progressive endurance, stimulating exercise as a means for post-heart attack therapy is gaining wide acceptance. Although a majority of post-heart attack rehabilitation efforts are helping patients to achieve a capacity to live a meaningful and active life, the major aim for control of heart disease should be prevention. Prevention should begin at birth through the formation of good nutritional and exercise habits. Dr. Per-Olaf Astrand, a famed Swedish Medical Doctor and Physiologist, asserts that because there is so much evidence that exercise can be beneficial to the functioning of the heart that we must seize the opportunity now to actively affect health in a positive way through a systematic improvement in physical fitness with training. He emphasizes that training the oxygen-transport system (the heart, lungs, and circulation) can be very important not only as a preventive measure but as a treatment for those unfortunate to be afflicted with atherosclerotic diseases of the circulation and heart.

## PHYSICAL ACTIVITY: A PREVENTIVE MEASURE
The American Heart Association's committee on exercise advocates physical activity "as an adjunct" to the control of blood pressure, blood lipid levels, and obesity. They caution against the supposition that exercise alone will prevent heart disease. However, they encourage exercise programs that are "tailored to the capacity and interest of the individual" for two reasons. They enrich the quality of life and, in combination with other measures (such as low-fat diets or eliminating smoking), they help reduce coronary risk. Physicians are increasingly aware of the possibilities of promoting and maintaining health through regular exercise. The American Medical Association's Committee on Exercise has declared, "Exercise is the most significant factor contributing to the health of the individual." The reasons are, by now, quite convincing.

### Population Studies
Studies have demonstrated a relationship between levels of physical activity and the incidence of coronary heart disease. The first study, and one of the largest, was done in London by Morris and his medical research team in 1953. They studied 30,000 men employed by the London Transit System, comparing inactive workers (the bus drivers) with active workers (the conductors who walk up and down the double-decker buses). They discov-

ered that the presumably less active bus drivers had many more coronaries than the more active conductors.

Morris followed this report by studying 10,000 London postal workers. Again, the active mail carriers had a lesser incidence of heart attacks than the inactive clerical workers. Dr. Ralph Paffenbarger of the University of California (Berkeley) recently reported on the results of a long-term study of almost 17,000 Harvard alumni. His findings suggest that heart attack risk can be significantly reduced by exercising—*but* only if the exercise is vigorous and burns substantial amounts of Calories. Paffenbarger found that those who exercise casually (burning fewer than 2000 Calories a week) ran a 64 percent greater heart attack risk than did their more active classmates (burning more than 2000 Calories a week). Vigorous activities such as swimming, running, handball, and cycling were cited by the California epidemiologist as the most desirable activities. These reports, although promising, must be viewed with caution. For example, the men with lower mortality may have possessed good cardiorespiratory systems that enable them to pursue the vigorous activities, rather than the activity developing the circulation to prevent a possible heart attack. Thus, these data in themselves only indicate an association of heart disease with inactivity, not necessarily a cause-and-effect relationship.

### The Irish Brothers Study
Recently, a nine-year study of 575 pairs of brothers born in Ireland was carried out by Harvard's School of Public Health and the School of Medicine at Trinity College, Dublin. One of each pair had remained in Ireland while the other had immigrated to the Boston area. The strictest scientific methods were employed to eliminate extraneous factors.

An astonishing conclusion was reached: the hearts of the Irishmen, whether rural or urban, were healthier than those of their Boston kinsmen. The Irish brothers had lower blood pressure and lower levels of cholesterol in their bloodstreams. The most astonishing fact was that the Irish brothers ate 400 to 500 more calories each day and had a higher percentage of animal fat in their daily diets than the Americans. Despite their diet, however, they weighed less, had less skinfold fat and, as mentioned, had lower cholesterol levels. The smoking and drinking habits of both were very similar. Then why were hearts of the Irish healthier than those of the American brothers? The results pointed directly to the fact that the Irish brothers were generally physically active while the Americans were generally sedentary. Physical activity, the researchers conclude, gave the Irish brothers their good health and good hearts.

**The Case for Exercise**
Coronary artery disease isn't like the measles; there is no protective vaccine you can take. It is disease that develops slowly and subtly. It is one of the dangers of living in a highly competitive but sedentary society. According to Dr. Sam Fox, a leading cardiologist, the data relating to physical activity and heart disease *suggest,* but fall short of proving, that an increase in habitual physical activity is beneficial. The most obvious benefits are in the area of improved quality of life, rather than necessarily in longevity. Dr. Fox recommends physical activity as a prudent means of enhancing health and improving the quality of one's life while also, probably, preventing coronary heart disease.

Vigorous exercise can be a very useful weapon against heart disease, but not by itself. Control of diet, blood pressure, blood fats, and tension, among other factors, are also important. Nevertheless, a well-organized, vigorous physical fitness program should be the focus of your efforts. Exercise is the positive approach. Instead of living a life of *don'ts*—don't eat this or that, don't become involved in tension-producing activities—exercise is a life of *do.* Rather than lead a life full of prohibitions, *do* exercise regularly and accentuate the positive way of life. Vigorous exercise will not only help

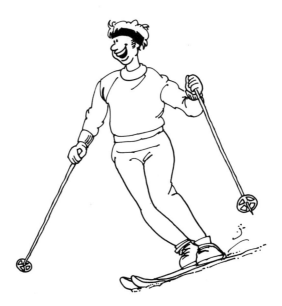

*In making regular exercise a habit you will be adding more "life to your years" and possibly "more years to your life."*

you to shed pounds of excess fat and keep them off, but it will also provide an ever-important outlet for the release of tension. Exercise can be a very effective means of controlling fatness, relieving tension, and normalizing other risk factors such as blood fats and blood pressure. In making regular exercise a habit, you will be adding more "life to your years" and possibly more "years to your life."

## KEY WORDS

ARTERIOSCLEROSIS: The advanced stage of atherosclerosis when the arteries become hardened.

ATHEROSCLEROSIS: The deposits and build-up of fatty substances on the inner walls of the arteries.

CHOLESTEROL: A waxy, fatty-like substance that serves an important role as a building block for formation of essential compounds vital to body functions. It is produced in the body and is also obtained by eating foods of animal origin. Elevated levels in the blood have been associated with an increased risk of heart and blood vessel disease.

CORONARY ARTERIES: The arteries that supply blood and nourishment to the heart muscle.

CORONARY HEART DISEASE: The impairment of the arteries of the heart (coronaries) from a build-up of cholesterol and associated fatty substances on the inner portion of the artery wall. See ATHERO-SCLEROSIS.

DIABETES: A chronic disorder of glucose (sugar) metabolism due to a disturbance of the normal insulin mechanism. See INSULIN.

DIASTOLIC PRESSURE: The lowest force exerted by the arterial blood flow against the walls of the vessels.

HYPERTENSION: Refers to a higher than normal blood pressure, usually defined as any systolic pressure above 140 mmHg and a diastolic pressure in excess of 90 mmHg.

INSULIN: A hormone that controls the rate of glucose entry into the cell.

LIPIDS: Fats, or fat-like substances such as fatty acids, triglyceride, and cholesterol.

LIPOPROTEIN: A type of protein that carries cholesterol and triglycerides in the bloodstream.

MYOCARDIAL INFARCTION: Heart attack or death of the heart muscle (myocardium) due to lack of oxygen.

OBESITY: An excessive amount of body fat or the state of being too fat.

SYSTOLIC PRESSURE: The greatest force exerted by the arterial blood flow against the walls of the vessels.

TRIGLYCERIDES: Fat particles that are stored in the body. They provide the main means for fat to be transported in the blood. Recent evidence has revealed an association with atherosclerosis.

TYPE A BEHAVIOR: The term used to describe people who exhibit an excessive competitive drive and time urgency. This behavior tends to predispose people to heart disease.

## SUPPLEMENTARY READINGS

Bassler, Thomas J., "Marathon Running and Immunity to Heart Disease." *The Physician and Sportsmedicine.* **3**: 77, April, 1975.

Blakeslee, Alton and Jeremiah Stamler, *Your Heart has Nine Lives.* Englewood Cliffs, New Jersey: Prentice-Hall, 1963.

Boyer, John L., "Heart Attack-Prevention Starts with Children." *Journal of Physical Education.* Special Edition: 103–105, March-April, 1972.

Dustin, Harriet P., "What Every Women Should Know About High Blood Pressure." *Family Health.* **7**:22, May, 1975.

Fox, Samuel III, John Naughton, and William Haskell, "Physical Activity and the Prevention of Coronary Heart Disease." *Annals of Clinical Research* **3**:404, 1971.

Friedman, Meyer and Ray H. Rosenman, *Type A Behavior and Your Heart.* Greenwich, Connecticut: Fawcett, 1974.

Golding, Lawrence, "Cholesterol and Exercise—A Ten Year Study." *Journal of Physical Education.* Special Edition: 106–110, March-April, 1972.

Graham, M.F., *Prescription For Life.* New York: David McKay Co., 1966.

Haskell, William, "Physical Activity and Heart Disease." *Journal of Physical Education.* Special Edition: 148–152, March-April, 1972.

Hellerstein, Herman, "Exercise and the Treatment of Heart Disease." *Journal of the South Carolina Medical Association* **65**:45, December, 1969.

Pollock, Michael, Jack Wilmore, and Samuel Fox III, *Health and Fitness Through Physical Activity.* New York: John Wiley & Sons, 1978.

Wilson, Phil (ed.), *Adult Fitness and Cardiac Rehabilitation.* Baltimore: University Park Press, 1975.

# chapter eleven

Sports participation can provide much enjoyment. Most people play sports for reasons other than health and sports provide meaningful experiences and challenges for them. Some sports may improve one's physical fitness somewhat. However, in general, to gain significant fitness benefits from your favorite sport, you need to be both highly skilled at it and to be able to devote many hours per week to playing it. Consider getting involved in the playing of one or more sports, especially those that are available in regard to cost, facilities, climate, and time. This chapter gives an overview of the many sports that can provide fun and fitness.

As you read this chapter give thought to the following statements:

• To imply that you can "play yourself" into good physical condition is lacking good research evidence. Most sports need to be supplemented with some basic conditioning to obtain a level of fitness that will enable you to better enjoy your play.

• The fitness benefits gained from sports participation vary from one person to the next. Such factors as your level of skill, intensity and dedication of participation, and the regularity in which you are able to play your chosen sport have much to do with the possible fitness benefits.

• Activities for developing and maintaining cardiorespiratory fitness must involve your total body in continuous and rhythmic exercise for a sustained period of time. Running, swimming, bicycling, and cross country skiing are good examples of lifetime sports that will provide a good stimulus for cardiorespiratory endurance. Sports such as tennis, raquetball, badminton, gymnastics, and ice skating, although somewhat intermittent, can also provide a good total body stimulus if played vigorously at a high level of skill.

• Quite often, people limit themselves in their sports selection. Many physical education programs in schools, colleges, and Y's now provide opportunities in a wide variety of activities. Consider taking instruction in some of these offerings and opening up new possibilities for a lifetime of enjoyable participation.

# a lifetime of sports participation

Throughout this book, we have described the physiological benefits of fitness. However, most of us need more reasons than physiological health to motivate us to exercise. It is not surprising to find that people who regularly jog, cycle, swim, or play sports do so because they enjoy it. The more interesting and meaningful an activity is, the greater our chance of involvement.

Because we all possess different personality structure and interests, we need to select sports and physical activities that are related to our own interests and desires. However, this is often easier said than done, simply because we lack adequate background for making a choice. The purpose of this chapter is to take a general look at a variety of sports activities that can add up to a lifetime of fun and fitness.

## A LOOK AT SPORTS AND PHYSICAL FITNESS

It is traditionally assumed that if you engage in a sport you will improve your level of physical fitness and, consequently, your general health. However, there is a wide difference among various sports in their contributions to physical fitness. Some sports, such as swimming and cycling, place great stress on the heart and lungs and help you to develop the function of these organs. Weight training helps you to increase strength and muscular endurance. Activities such as karate or gymnastics contribute more to flexibility and strength than do bowling and archery. The physical fitness contributions of different sports are varied and, in some cases, very specific and limited.

For years many physical educators, coaches, and even athletes have operated under the mistaken notion that you can "play yourself" into good physical condition. This thesis sounds reasonable, but we now know that basic conditioning is needed to supplement most sports programs. The idea is that you should condition yourself first to better enjoy your play. You have to be reasonably fit to get the maximum benefit from your chosen sport.

It is easy to get bored with jogging on a track or swimming laps in a pool. But anyone active in sports finds these activities reasonable when combined with favorite sports. Whatever your preference—tennis, scuba diving, skiing, or schoolyard basketball—you will enjoy these activities more if you keep your body in firm muscular shape and in good cardiorespiratory health through a program of fitness training. Most likely you can't play at your favorite sport every day, or even three or four days a week. It is wise to keep in shape in the intervals, not only for your general health, but also to provide a more rewarding experience when you do get a chance to play.

## LIFETIME SPORTS

In the following pages we describe some popular sporting activities to help you choose one or several that are most suitable to you for a lifetime of fitness. It is impossible to discuss all sports with the limits of this chapter. But most of the ones we discuss here (with the exception of golf, bowling, and archery) provide good vigorous activity. Organized team sports, such as basketball, field hockey, soccer, and volleyball, although very vigorous and enjoyable, have not been included. This is not meant to deny the importance of regular play on a varsity, sports club, or intramural team. But team sports require facilities and organization beyond the reach of most people. This chapter emphasizes individual and dual sports. Now is the time to begin developing skills and interests in sports that can be readily played in the years to come. A wide variety of interests should be encouraged, and this is the purpose of lifetime sports. All of these activities are exciting and challenging, and all possess the qualities that make a sport enjoyable and popular. Most of them are suitable for people of all ages.

Each description is written with the assumption that the reader has little first-hand knowledge of the activity. Each sport is briefly described. The physical fitness requirements and potential benefits from regular play are indicated. We know that the benefits from sports participation will vary from one person to the next, and any attempt to rate and compare the sports as to their relative contribution for developing physical fitness can be questioned. To date the research to support such judgment is limited. Nevertheless, at the end of this chapter, we have devised some charts that rate the various lifetime sports on their relative worth for developing and maintaining physical fitness.

### Alpine Skiing

Descending a snow-covered slope on skis can be a vigorous and challenging adventure. The popularity of this winter sport has been steadily growing, because of improved methods of instruction and the spread of ski

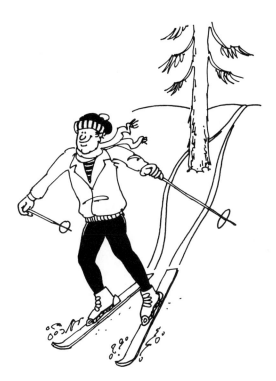

*Alpine skiing*

resorts. Snow machines have now made skiing possible even where winters are mild.

The physical requirements of the recreational skier differ, of course, from those of the competitive racer, but some needs are quite basic. For the turns and maneuvers that the sport requires, every skier must have a good strength and endurance in the leg muscles. For this reason, ski instructors recommend regular conditioning of these muscles before and during the ski season. When your legs tire easily on the slopes, you are vulnerable to accident. Although cardiorespiratory fitness doesn't seem to be a vital requirement for the recreational skier, efficient functioning of the heart and lungs certainly is advantageous if you intend repeated runs down the slopes. As usual, the level of your skiing ability and the vigor with which you ski determines the fitness benefits.

Downhill skiing can be hazardous. Thus, reliable equipment, observance of safety precautions, and sound instruction are necessary. This sport demands well-developed form and technique. It is recommended that you master the fundamentals before taking any risks. Learning how to stop, turn, and even fall properly are the basis for the first lessons. You must then learn to maintain your balance and control your downhill speed. Most ski resorts provide certified ski instruction. The most widespread of the new teaching systems is the *graduated length method,* in which skiers start on four-foot skis, move on to five-footers, and finally to regular-length skis, all within a week or so of ski instruction.

Alpine skiing is expensive. Besides warm ski clothing, you will need skis, boots, bindings, and poles. This equipment makes for a very costly package. Normally, as a beginner, you should rent equipment until you have more knowledge of the sport. Then you can make wise decisions when you begin to outfit yourself. Skis, boots, and poles can be rented at most ski resorts at a cost of $5 to $10 a day. A group lesson will cost around four dollars an hour. However, when you stay at a resort on a five-day or weekend package plan, your lessons and tow fee are quite often included with your lodging and meals.

**Archery**
Archery calls for precision of movement, and muscular force is needed in drawing the bowstring. As a result, the sport requires strength and some endurance in the muscles of the shoulder, upper and lower arm, and abdomen. It differs from most of the activities in this chapter, however, because it is static: little movement is required beyond that needed for aiming. Obviously, the physical fitness requirements and benefits of archery are very limited. Still, a serious competitor would be wise to follow an exercise program that develops strength, muscular endurance, and cardiorespiratory endurance. Such training would reduce the possibility of muscle fatigue.

A typical bow ranges from five to six feet in length. Bows vary according to the number of pounds of pull required to draw the arrow to its full length. This figure is referred to as the *weight* of the bow. Normally women start with a 25- to 30-pound bow, while men can usually handle a 30- to 35 pound bow. As your skill and strength improve, you then progress to a heavier bow, which increases your accuracy in aiming. Bows are generally made of either lemonwood or fiberglass. Some archers use a finger tab or shooting glove to protect the hand that touches the bowstring. Also, an arm guard for the bow arm, usually made of leather, should be used to protect the forearm from injury. The cost of outfitting yourself with a bow can range

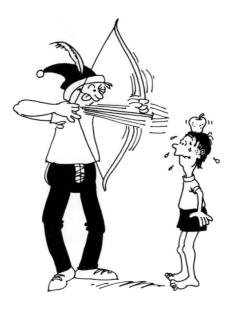

*Archery*

from around $10 for a solid fiberglass instructional bow to more deluxe models (designed for competition or hunting) in the $100 range. Target arrows can be purchased for about a half-dollar each, whereas hunting arrows cost about three times as much.

The standard archery target has four rings around a bull's-eye. Scoring ranges from one point for hitting the outside white ring to nine points for an arrow in the bull's-eye. In a tournament, a prescribed number of arrows are shot from various distances and the scores are added.

Through the ages, archery has been practiced for both hunting and warfare. Today it is a skilled sport with many devotees. Frequent tournaments provide opportunities for competition.

### Backpacking and Camping

Hiking into the back country symbolizes for many people a return to the basics. Everyone feels some exhiliration in viewing a sunrise in the wilderness, watching a sparking campfire, or breathing the air in a pine-scented forest. The backpacker can attain a feeling of complete freedom that perhaps no other sport provides. Backpacking is an unregulated sport, too, for there are no formal rules and no required levels of skill. It can be done

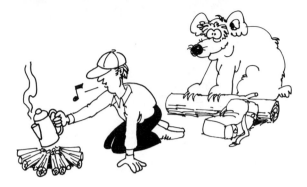

*Backpacking and camping*

alone or with friends. It can be carried out in all extremes of temperature, altitude, and terrain.

Obviously a good level of physical fitness is a boon. On occasion you may have to draw on your reserves of strength to continue up a trail or to complete the trek to your planned destination for the day. Precisely how much energy you will require will depend on the terrain, your body size, your walking speed, and the size of your backpack. For instance, walking in snow is more demanding than walking on a level footpath. Also, more energy is required for a 220-lb person than for a 120-lb person over the same terrain. In short, backpacking can be relatively mild, or it can be very demanding.

The beginner should make careful plans and follow a well-marked trail. It is also a good idea to have an experienced guide along. There are several organizations that promote backpacking and camping expeditions for people of all levels of experience. The Sierra Club (San Francisco) and the Appalachian Mountain Club (Boston) are two of the most popular. Such organizations run instructional clinics and publish information.

Planned hikes can eliminate much of the uncertainty of backpacking. You should have instruction in planning your trip and in outdoor food preparation. Suitable clothing (footwear, rain gear, and insulated garments) also needs careful attention.

The feasibility of backpacking as a sport is influenced by the area you live, the time of year, the climate, and your own abilities. With a proper background in backpacking skills, a good level of physical fitness, and the availability of a hiking area, you can enjoy the great outdoors to the fullest. Whatever your aspirations, backpacking can be adapted to meet your desires.

## Badminton

Badminton is a popular racquet game that consists of batting a plastic or feathered *shuttle* back and forth over a net. So long as they are well matched, even beginners can generate much competitive excitement. To produce fitness benefits, however, badminton needs to be played skillfully and vigorously (not as it is practiced in most backyards). Researchers at the University of California, Santa Barbara, studied the intensities of various sports as played by young women of above-average skill. Badminton was ranked as a moderate-energy-cost activity. However, the energy cost depends on the vigor and duration of play.

Badminton requires quick starts and stops, powerful smashes, drives, clears, and drops. As a result, to play regularly, you need a good level of muscular strength and endurance in the arms and legs and an adequate cardiorespiratory fitness. Good hand to eye coordination is also essential. Coaches of the sport state that to play winning badminton, you must develop endurance along with the appropriate strokes. Running, cycling, and skipping rope are good endurance activities; weight training exercises for

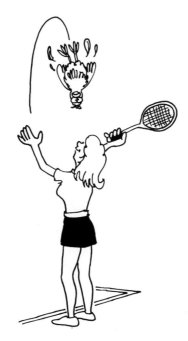

*Badminton*

the hand and forehand will strengthen the whip of the wrist at impact, which gives explosive force to your shots.

The principal items of equipment you will need are a racquet, a few shuttles, a net, and a pair of rubber-soled tennis shoes. There is a wide range of quality in badminton equipment. Racquets vary from under $10.00 to around $40.00 for the top model. Gut-strung racquets are better than nylon, but nylon wears longer. The shuttlecocks or *birds* are made from cork or rubber and goose feathers, but plastic birds are now on the market and are very durable. A can of six shuttlecocks costs around $5.00.

Essentially, badminton is an indoor game. Most gymnasiums have badminton court lines painted on the floor. However, the main problem is finding out when these facilities are available. Whether played as a doubles or singles game, badminton requires a wide variety of shots and much strategy.

### Bicycling

Bicycling provides wholesome fun for all ages. Vigorous, sustained cycling makes strong demands on the cardiorespiratory system. However, there is more to bicycling than just good exercise. The cyclist enjoys the camaraderie of touring and the pleasures of the countryside.

In general, we can classify bicycling into five categories: transportation, touring, racing, physical fitness training, and moderate recreation. For some people, a bike is a weekend plaything, while for others it provides daily transportation. Leisurely pedaling will not benefit your fitness, but vigorous and sustained pedaling can stimulate your lungs, heart, and muscles adequately for fitness gains. Racing requires a high level of physical fitness

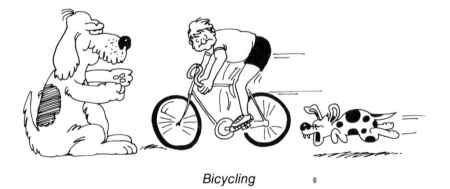

Bicycling

and many hours of riding (conditioning) are necessary to compete. Most of us do not wish to race, but touring and vigorous pleasure riding can contribute to our overall fitness. Naturally, the tempo of riding will govern the benefits. In general, riding at a four-to-five-minute mile tempo for a good 30- to 45-minute workout will provide adequate training for the cardiorespiratory system.

Cycle touring is becoming more popular each year. These trips involve one-day or weekend jaunts or longer tours. They can be combined with camping, but gear must be kept to a minimum (a lightweight tent, a sleeping bag, and cooking apparatus). Your route and equipment need to be planned in detail, and you will need a good bicycle with at least 10 gear speeds. Be sure in advance that each day's journey is within your physical capacity, and try to travel with a group or an experienced leader. The American Youth Hostels schedules bicycle tours from most major cities; joining an AYH chapter in your area would be a wise decision if you wish to tour seriously. Most cycling books give detailed information on other cycling groups.

To discuss all the aspects of bicycle racing would take a chapter in itself. In some European countries, bicycle racing is a national sport and professionals can make a good deal of money. The kinds of races vary from team to individual, from long-distance to sprints, from time trials to mass events, and from road to indoor racing. In the United States, the Amateur Bicycle League of America is the governing body of racing.

In reality, touring and racing are two absolutely different types of cycling. Racing requires tremendous physical training and competitive skill; cycling is simply a healthful hobby. But whether you use a bike to get from home to work and back each day, or for weekend touring trips, the bicycle can be an excellent and enjoyable means of staying fit.

## Bowling

The first record of bowling in America goes back to 1623, when Dutch settlers introduced the game to Manhattan; today it is still prospering. According to its promoters, bowling is now the most popular participation sport in America. However, although it requires good rhythm and coordination, bowling is only a mild exercise with little physical fitness benefits. Research established years ago that bowling in a foursome requires only about twice the energy it takes to sit in a chair. The reason is that about 80 to 90 percent of the time, you are simply sitting and watching the others in your group bowl.

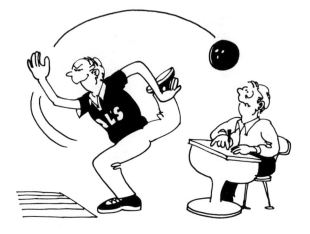

*Bowling*

Bowling leagues can be found at all bowling centers. It is probably this type of competition, along with a handicap system that allows people of varying abilities to compete on an equal basis, that makes the sport popular. You do not have to purchase any equipment to bowl. The bowling alley provides the balls, and bowling shoes can be rented at a nominal fee. If you become a serious bowler you will most likely buy your own ball. In this way you become accustomed to using the same ball each time you bowl. The fee charged for using the lanes varies, but when compared to the fees charged for other sports, it is very reasonable.

## Canoeing and Kayaking

Canoeing is a sport with a rich heritage. It originated centuries ago as a mode of travel in the wilderness, where passage on foot was difficult. The birch canoes of the Indians and explorers are familiar from American history. For devotees, canoeing brings a sense of freedom and a retreat to a simple life.

Although many people think of canoeing as a quiet activity associated with the pleasures of fishing and camping, it can be very strenuous. When performed as an Olympic sport, canoeing requires good cardiorespiratory fitness and a high level of muscular strength and endurance in the arms, shoulders, and trunk. At the camping and touring level, however, the main requirement is strength and endurance in the arms and shoulders. Daily canoeing can develop the muscles of the arms, shoulders, and back.

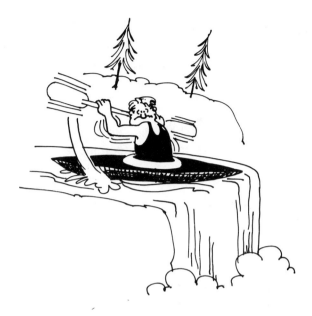

*Canoeing and kayaking*

White-water canoeing, racing, and kayaking are related activities for people with competitive interests. A kayak sits low in the water, and the top is covered except for the cockpit where the paddler sits; the paddle is double-bladed. Kayaks are built for racing or touring and for flat water or rapids. As in canoeing, muscular strength and endurance are prerequisites, and good reflexes and skills are necessary for maneuvering the boat. Cardiorespiratory fitness is also a necessary ingredient for the demands of paddling.

Instruction in all phases of canoeing and boating is readily available at numerous national aquatic schools conducted annually by the American Red Cross Water Safety Service, summer camps, and local recreation areas. A prerequisite for all potential canoeists is an ability to swim comfortably in deep water. The American Canoe Association promotes recreational canoeing. This organization also sponsors national competition and has full responsibility for conducting Olympic trials.

Canoes vary in size and shape. The most popular lengths are from 15 to 17 feet. They are made out of wood, fiberglass, or the most durable material, aluminum. The cost of a standard-sized aluminum canoe runs under $500. Many enthusiasts rent from commercial canoe liveries, which are quite common near large streams and waterways throughout the country. Rentals are paid for by the hour or by the destination. Trucks transport you and the canoe to a starting destination and pick you up at a designated spot downstream.

## Cross-Country Skiing

Cross-country skiing (often called Nordic skiing) is a national sport in the Scandinavian countries and is rapidly becoming a popular recreational sport in the United States. Nordic skiing is generally divided into two categories, touring and competitive racing. Touring is much the less strenuous, as the skiers travel at their own pace on quiet trails throughout the countryside and forests. In racing, the pressure of competition demands great muscular stamina, cardiorespiratory endurance, and athletic skill. Competitive cross-country skiers, male and female, have some of the highest fitness levels in the world.

Cross-country skiing can be learned in a very short time. According to some instructors, beginners can learn the fundamentals of the kick-and-glide and poling during the first lesson; enjoyment is well within the reach of most people. In the kick-and-glide technique, the skier uses both a kicking action of the legs and a poling action of the arms to propel the body forward.

The intensity of your skiing is just as variable as that of jogging. Your exercise work load is determined by the difficulty of the terrain, your pace,

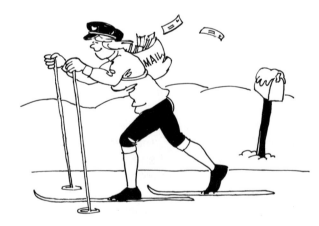

*Cross-country skiing*

and the length of the rest periods you take. If you can ski with vigor, you will provide a good training stimulus for your heart and lungs and total body musculature. Habitual joggers and cyclists who live in cold-winter regions find cross-country skiing a refreshing activity during the snowy season.

Ski touring can be done anywhere there is snow. Golf courses, logging trails, park trails, and open fields make fine areas for winter skiing. Many ski resorts are now catering to cross-country ski enthusiasts as well by maintaining special marked touring trails and offering instruction in cross-country skiing. Sporting goods stores and ski shops quite often sponsor cross-country ski clinics.

The equipment for cross-country skiing is rather inexpensive when compared to that for alpine skiing. Touring boots, bindings, skis, and poles cost only a third of their downhill equivalents. Most ski resorts will rent complete equipment for under ten dollars a day. If you have snowy winters and enjoy the outdoors, ski touring offers many benefits.

## Dance

Dancing is included in this chapter because it can require a complete use of every muscle in the body. Modern dance (contemporary dance) requires good muscle elasticity along with controlled movements; it generally demands greater muscular strength, endurance, and flexibility than other kinds of dance. The warm-ups, exercises, and techniques of this kind of

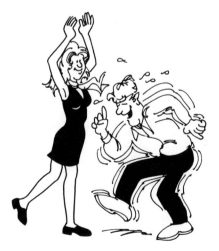

*Dance*

dancing are excellent activities for general body conditioning and tone. As usual, the intensity, duration, and frequency of your practice and dance periods determine the benefits. Regular and vigorous modern dance can be a very good fitness activity. In addition, the serious dancer experiences a release of emotional and mental tension through strenuous self-expression.

Social dances, as well as square and folk dancing, are largely confined to exercise of the legs and feet. Again, some forms of these dances can be quite vigorous, expecially folk dances. However, few people dance intensely enough to realize significant cardiorespiratory development. Most forms of social dancing are of low to moderate intensity.

Instruction in dance is widely available. Many private dance studios are listed in the yellow pages, and public adult education programs, YM/YWCAs, and colleges offer many forms of dance instruction.

### Distance Running

Today, there are thousands of dedicated distance runners who run not only for the obvious health benefits, but for personal pleasure and the fun of competition. Regular daily workouts place an invigorating stress on your cardiorespiratory system. Running is one of the best exercises for developing and maintaining physical fitness. And anyone can run; the sport does not require the highly developed motor skills that many sports demand. For most distance runners, winning road races is not the dominant objective. In fact, many people run regularly all of their lives without entering a race.

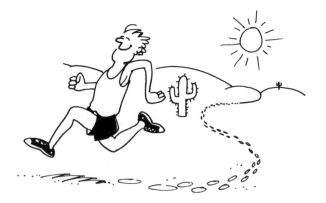

*Distance running*

Competitive races for men and women of various ages and levels of fitness are staged on a regular basis throughout the country. Running clubs and jogging associations sponsor such events on the local, state, and regional level. *Runner's World,* a magazine devoted to running enthusiasts, lists many of the upcoming regional and national road races in each issue.

Although token fees are charged for entry into most races, running is a relatively inexpensive sport. The serious runner has no problem finding suitable terrain to run on; streets, parking lots, or footpaths will do. Durable running shoes are the main expense. Good-quality jogging or running shoes with cushioned heels can be fitted at most sporting goods stores. Even though name-brand shoes cost over $20, proper footwear is a must to protect your feet and to avoid injuries to your joints.

## Fencing

The object of the sport fencing is not to inflict injury but to demonstrate an ability to outmaneuver your opponent. The combatants wear protective clothing, and the sword blades are flexible and blunted for safety.

Fencing requires stamina and wrist strength to hold the sword up continuously. Quick reactions, speed, and good coordination are all essential for success. In early fencing drills repeated lunging and recovering helps to

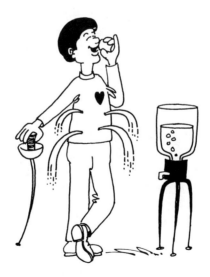

*Fencing*

condition the arms and legs. Because of the nature of the movements of this sport, however, it cannot be classified as a good cardiorespiratory developer. World-class fencers have high aerobic capacities, but they train for it; they also do high-speed interval training to develop their anaerobic fitness. The "winded" feeling one can get from vigorous fencing is not necessarily an aerobic response. Most likely it is anaerobic, stemming from the high intensity but short duration of the fencing movements.

The three basic weapons are the foil, epée, and saber. The foil is used by beginners and is the only one used by women. It is the lightest of the three weapons and doesn't require as much arm strength. Relatively speaking, fencing equipment is inexpensive and durable. In addition to a foil, you will need protective equipment. This includes a strong mask, a padded white jacket, and a padded fencing glove for the sword hand.

In learning to fence your main emphasis should be on sound fundamentals. The en-garde position, the lunge, and the retreat (recovery from the lunge), must be learned at the start; thereafter you can advance into various more complicated attacks and defenses. Instruction in fencing is not as readily available as in other individual sports. Fencing clubs for men and women are found in most of the large metropolitan areas, and they often provide some instruction. However, most fencers get their start in college physical education programs. The Amateur Fencing League of America organizes all fencing tournaments in the United States. Divisions have been established for local competition that eventually lead to national championship events for a highly skilled performer.

## Golf

Arnold Palmer once wrote:

*Golf is deceptively simple and endlessly complicated. A child can play it well, and a grown man can never master it. Any single round of it is full of unexpected triumphs and seemingly perfect shots that end in disaster. It is almost a science, yet it is a puzzle without an answer. It is gratifying and tantalizing, precise and unpredictable; it requires complete concentration and total relaxation. It satisfies the soul and frustrates the intellect. It is at the same time rewarding and maddening–and it is without doubt the greatest game mankind has ever invented.*[1]

[1]Arnold Palmer, *Sports Illustrated,* "My Game and Yours," July 15, 1963.

This unique description indicates why golf has so many devoted participants. As practiced by professionals, it is a highly skilled sport. However, a
little instruction and a few rounds of play are all that are required to make
golf an enjoyable outdoor recreation for the average man or woman.

Reasonable perfection of the golf swing takes considerable practice;
strength is necessary for powerful and consistent shots. However, the actual play of golf doesn't require any substantial cardiorespiratory endurance. The caloric cost of golf has been determined by research, and it is
only about three times the energy required for sitting in a chair. This low
energy demand points up the unsuitability of golf as a physical fitness
stimulus for the body. Golf courses average about four or five miles in
length. However, because of the constant standing and watching, the golfer
is actually walking only a third of his total time on the course. According to a
University of Illinois study in 1965, sedentary men showed no changes in
cardiorespiratory fitness after a full season of golf. Their cardiorespiratory
fitness was greatly inferior to that of a similar group of men who exercised
regularly in a jogging program.

The fact that golf is not a suitable physical fitness activity does not mean
that it is worthless, however; golf offers an enjoyable diversion from the
everyday routine in a pleasant outdoor setting. Hitting a good tee shot down
the middle of the fairway, stopping an iron shot close to the flag stick, or
curling in a 20 foot putt can be a gratifying experience.

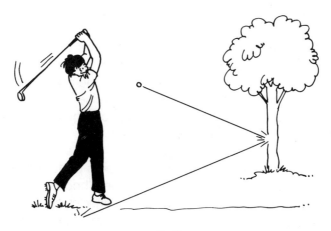

Golf

Golf is one of the more expensive sports, and poor equipment can certainly interfere with progress in learning the game. Clubs can be rented for a nominal fee at most golf course pro shops. However, after becoming familiar with the game, you may wish to buy your own. Golf equipment is sold in all sporting goods stores, but usually a golf professional's shop is the best place to buy them. The golf pro carries top-quality equipment, and normally he will allow you to try the clubs out on a driving range before you buy them. A set of high-quality clubs can run well beyond $400, but an adequate starter set (a partial set) can be purchased for under $100. Used sets will be even cheaper. Golf shoes cost over $20, and official golf balls can be bought for around a dollar each. Accessories, such as golf carts, umbrellas, and gloves can further increase your expenditure. Green fees can run anywhere from $3 for 18 holes up to as much as $10 on some championship courses. Many golf courses offer seasonal memberships, which are decidedly cheaper if you are going to be playing regularly. Instruction by a qualified teaching professional is strongly recommended.

## Gymnastics

For decades, gymnastics has been one of the most popular sports in many European nations, and it is now one of the fastest growing sports in the United States. It is both challenging and satisfying, and, when compared with other activities for all-around development, it rates very high.

Regular, strenuous participation in gymnastic routines will result in worthy physical fitness effects. As always, of course, these benefits are directly related to the intensity and regularity of one's participation. In gymnastics you are constantly working against your body weight, stimulating the major muscles of the entire body. Gymnastics enhances agility, balance, coordination, muscular endurance, strength, and flexibility. It provides long-lasting values such as good muscle tone and development, and a trim and flexible body. Continuous floor exercise is the best activity for cardiorespiratory development. For the advanced gymnast a supplementary running program would be advantageous.

A form of gymnastics intended especially for women is emerging, called *modern gymnastics*. It entails natural movements performed continuously with or without supplements such as balls, ropes, hoops, and Indian clubs. These activities are executed to music. Some universities and YM/YWCAs are now teaching these routines along with the standard gymnastic activities involving tumbling, the side horse, parallel bars, horizontal bar, rings, and floor exercises.

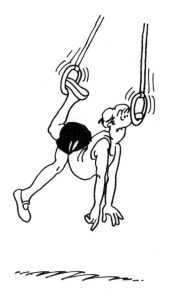

*Gymnastics*

Competition is available for the serious gymnastic performer. Meets for senior and junior men and women are sponsored at the district and national level. Information can be obtained from gymnastic instructors in your area. School competition at the high school and intercollegiate level is quite popular.

### Handball

Handball is played on an enclosed, four-walled court, although there are variations of the game suitable for one- to three-walled courts. It may be played by two (singles), three ("cut throat"), or four players (doubles). The object is to hit a hard rubber ball against the front wall in such a way that it bounces twice on the floor before one's opponent can return it. Strategy involves using all the walls of the court as well as the ceiling. Positioning is an important skill of the sport.

The entire body is involved in playing handball. Both arms are used to deliver the force to the ball, and the legs must move quickly. The heart and lungs are extensively stressed. The handball player needs a very high level of motor skill and intense concentration. This strenuous and exciting sport far surpasses many other forms of physical activity for attaining and main-

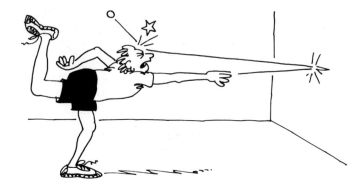

*Handball*

taining good physical condition. Of course, the skill of the participants and the vigor with which the game is played will determine the benefits. Using handball as your sole physical fitness program is not recommended. However, you need better-than-average cardiorespiratory fitness to perform adequately. Many serious handballers jog to supplement their regular handball play. You should prepare yourself physically for play with general stretching, strength, and flexibility exercises.

Physical size or sex are not limiting factors in handball (unless you are fat). The sport is especially popular in colleges and universities, in YM/YWCAs, and in many private athletic clubs, and competitive tournaments are quite common. Generally they are set up for all levels of skill. The only equipment needed aside from gym wear is a pair of leather gloves and the official black rubber ball. If court facilities are available, the cost of this sport is minimal.

## Ice Skating

Ice skating has always been a popular sport for people of all ages and levels of skill. Thanks to indoor arenas, it is now being enjoyed by more people than ever. For some skaters, gliding over the ice on a rink or pond is enjoyment enough. For others, figure skating or dancing patterns to music offers a rewarding challenge. Still other skaters play ice hockey or race.

In general, all forms of ice skating tax the major muscle groups of the arms, legs, abdomen, and back. Good muscle tone and flexibility are positive benefits from regular skating. If the skating is strenuous enough, the

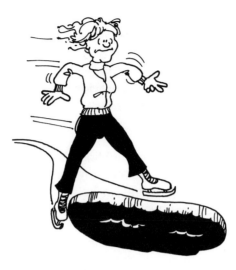

*Ice skating*

cardiorespiratory system will also be stressed. Though figure skating is normally only of moderate intensity, unless you are highly skilled, the sport of speed skating is a very demanding activity.

Figure skating combines grace, daring, precision, stamina, and endurance. The United States Figure Skating Association (USFSA), the governing body of amateur figure skating on ice, sanctions various events for its members and sponsors official tests. There are programs of instruction for all levels of skill, and competitions on every level give skaters an incentive to improve their proficiency. Sectional and national championships lead to international competitions. Obviously, competitive success requires many hours of dedicated practice and superior coordination and conditioning. However, most figure skaters in the United States who belong to the USFSA member clubs skate simply because they enjoy the sport.

Speed skating, by contrast, is aimed at covering a specified distance in the shortest period of time. The fast starts and powerful strokes of speed skating require a greater intensity of effort than does figure skating and, thus, greater physiological fitness.

Skates of average quality cost from $20 to $40 but top-quality equipment can run as much as $150. Proper fitting is extremely important. As a rule, your skates should be at least one size smaller than your regular shoe size.

You should wear one pair of light wool socks and be sure that your skates are laced properly. Having "weak ankles" is a poor reason for not skating; generally, ankle problems are a result of poorly fitted skates.

Proper instruction will help you progress to many hours of enjoyable skating. Generally local skating clubs provide the best teaching. The cost of group or individual lessons is variable.

## Judo

Judo is a method of bare-handed fighting developed by the Japanese, matching two people in a well regulated and highly disciplined contest. Its original intent was largely defensive, unlike other systems of combat. This sport provides both not only physical but also mental challenges.

Judo training concentrates on teaching throwing techniques and grappling skills. This repetitious practice of the art of throwing and grappling requires muscular strength and endurance, balance, agility, and coordination. In addition, there are exercises for proper falling to enable you to withstand the forces in being thrown. Traditionally, the physical training is also ·used to obtain moral and spiritual goals. Mastery of the techniques requires considerable practice and dedication.

Judo competition provides opportunities to test your own skills against those of an unfamiliar opponent. But the emphasis is on art and skill rather than brute force. The time limit of judo bouts is usually between three and ten minutes. A point is awarded for a forceful and clean throw, a hold down, or a lock. All activities are conducted within the mat area.

The United States Judo Federation recognizes specific levels of skill,

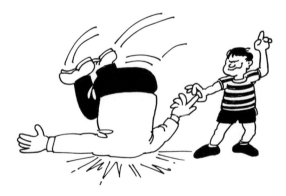

*Judo*

symbolized by the color of belt you wear. A white belt is awarded to the beginner; there are three degrees of brown belt for skilled beginners, and then the well-known black belt for the expert. Promotions to the various ranks in Judo are achieved by study, tournaments, and examinations in which you must demonstrate the physical skills and pass written and oral tests.

Competent judo instruction can often be found in the YM/YWCAs in most cities. Many colleges and schools also now offer instruction. Although judo can be practiced out of doors, it is usually practiced indoors with adequate padding and mats to prevent injury. The judo uniform of *gi* can be purchased for less than twenty dollars.

## Karate

Karate is an offensive and defensive martial art using both the fists and the feet through arm thrusts and kicks. It has been described as the most violent method of unarmed self defense known to man. Because of the potential dangers in practicing this form of combat, it is imperative that you learn the proper techniques from a qualified and certified instructor. When properly practiced and supervised, however, karate can be a safe and enjoyable sport. Community YM/YWCAs, many colleges, and some high schools now offer karate instruction. Private exercise halls (called dojos) are also quite common in many metropolitan areas.

During a competitive match, it is a violation to strike vital parts of your opponent directly because of the possibility of serious injury. Points are

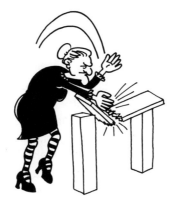

Karate

awarded by referees who judge the execution of the various movements. One scores by achieving a position from which it is possible to strongly thrust into a vital part of the opponent; the thrust must be stopped just before the point of contact.

Training in the necessary movements such as strikes, thrusts, kicks, and parries is vigorous. The physical training focuses on the development of stance, movements, balance, speed, timing, and breathing. There are two basic types of training. One is to practice the movements without an opponent; the other is free sparring with an opponent. Preparatory exercises strengthen and limber the joints as well as the muscles; most of these warmup routines bear some relation to the actual karate techniques. The actual exercises consist of hundreds of repetitions of each particular strike, kick, or block.

Drilling in karate involves the development of muscular strength and endurance and puts much emphasis on flexibility and coordination. Karate practice will not improve your cardiorespiratory endurance; you must supplement it with some form of jogging, running, or similar training.

A pajamalike white cotton garment, called a *gi,* is the standard karate apparel. In addition, a colored belt that denotes the wearer's official rank is worn around the waist and tied in front. Throughout the world, promotions in rank are achieved by demonstrated skills and knowledge, with the level of skill indicated by the color of the belt. There are 10 non-black-belt ranks (white, yellow, green, brown) that must first be obtained before one graduates to the black-belt ranks, which also number 10.

## Orienteering

Orienteering originated in Sweden, where it is a national sport with mass participation. A weekend of orienteering in Sweden might draw two to three thousand or more participants. In the United States its popularity has increased steadily in the past few years; the first U.S. Orienteering Championships were held at Southern Illinois University in 1970.

Orienteering is a form of cross-country running that makes use of a map and compass to guide the participants through an unknown countryside. It is a combination of hiking, climbing, running, jogging, and walking. A detailed topographical map presents the terrain of the area in exact terms, including all streams, ponds, paths, forests, marshes, meadows, fences, buildings, and land contours. The compass helps the orienteer to find a bearing in the fields and forests.

On the map of the area, control stations are indicated by small red

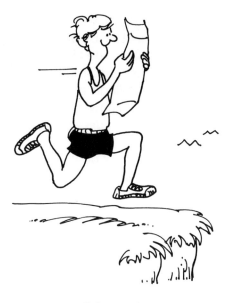

*Orienteering*

circles. These circles designate markers, usually small red and white flags, which have been placed on the ground in a fixed sequence. The flags cannot be seen from any previous station and generally are not visible from more than 20 to 30 yards away. Thus the orienteer must use the map and compass to find them. The runners begin from the starting point at one-minute intervals. The object is to progress as rapidly as possible to the various control stations in the sequence marked on the map. At each station the runner punches his card with a special punch found at the station. The stations must be reached in the designated order. The person who negotiates the course in the quickest time is the winner.

Orienteering demands accurate map reading, sound decisions (sometimes the shortest route between two points is not always the best), and a high level of cardiorespiratory fitness. Because you sprint on open terrain, run up hills, and scurry through thick forests, you must be in excellent physical condition to perform well. Perfecting your map-reading and compass skills will also help to reduce your time. The ability to make quick decisions about which route to travel is a skill that comes only with experience.

Orienteering is an inexpensive activity. All you need are running shoes and an adequate orienteering compass, with a transparent protractor plate, which costs about five dollars. Most clubs or sponsors of meets charge a registration fee of around five dollars. The United States Orienteering Federation promotes clinics and workshops around the country and sanctions the championship competitions. College physical education departments often have information about upcoming workshops and competitions.

### Racquetball

Racquetball combines some of the best qualities of squash and handball. It is a sport that most people can play with reasonable success after brief instruction and practice.

It is played indoors in a four-walled rectangular court with a ceiling 20 feet high. Equipment includes a short handle, tennislike racquet and a soft rubber ball, slightly smaller than a tennis ball. Clothing, such as tennis shoes, socks, shorts, and T-shirt, is the customary dress. The initial investment for racquetball is quite reasonable. Good metal or fiberglass composite racquets start at 15 dollars. The balls come two to a can for about 3 to 4 dollars.

Racquetball is a demanding sport and provides a very good workout. It requires arm, shoulder, and wrist strength and great agility. In addition, its fast competitive pace demands training, and cardiorespiratory endurance

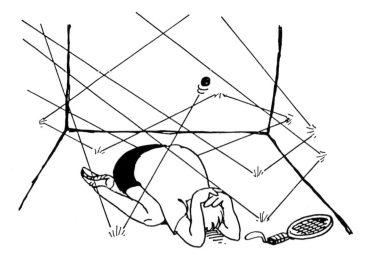

*Racquetball*

is needed for continued play. Played hard, this sport can certainly contribute to cardiorespiratory fitness. It is suggested that you try a supplemental program of endurance training (e.g.; jogging and cycling) along with practice in racquetball itself. Expertise at racquetball is as much a matter of reflexes as of overall technique.

## Scuba Diving

Scuba diving opens up a strange and mysterious underwater world. The scuba diver has all the standard equipment of a skin diver—mask, fins, and so on—plus a tank of air that makes it possible to stay under water for exploration; scuba is an acronym for Self-Contained Underwater Breathing Apparatus. Underwater exploration can be exciting, and the physical illusion of weightlessness is a refreshing experience. Many scuba enthusiasts develop additional diving interests such as spear fishing, photography, and scientific study.

Scuba diving will not contribute to physical fitness because your movements underwater have to be slow and easy, and hard exertion can deplete your air supply. However, a high fitness capacity *can* help you, because you will not require as much air as a poorly conditioned diver does. In other words, the better your cardiorespiratory fitness, the longer you will be able to remain under water and enjoy your dive. Training by swimming regularly would be most advantageous. However, if a swimming area is not readily

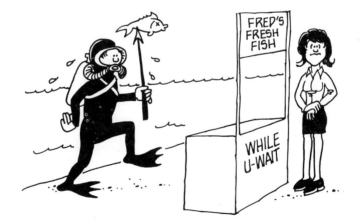

*Scuba diving*

available, a general conditioning program of jogging and calisthenic exercise will suffice.

Proper instruction is a must for any beginner. The thrills of scuba diving are tempered by the hazards. Most diving accidents are the result not of equipment failure, but of a lack of knowledge, skill, or training. Thus it is absolutely essential to take a scuba course from a certified instructor who can systematically expose you to the basics of the sport. Many schools, colleges, swim clubs, YM/YWCAs, recreation departments, and camps now offer such courses. Membership in an accredited diving group assures you of regular sessions that are well-organized and supervised.

Standard apparatus includes a face mask, swim fins, and a compressed air cylinder with airhose and regulator. In addition, in all but the warmest of waters, you will need a rubberized wetsuit. The cost of such equipment can run anywhere from $500 to $1000. Although expensive, with proper care the equipment will last a long time.

**Skin Diving**
Skin diving, as opposed to scuba diving, is underwater swimming without breathing equipment. The only equipment in skin diving is a pair of swim

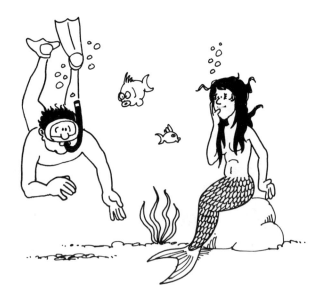

*Skin diving*

fins, a glass face mask, and a snorkel tube for surface breathing. The snorkel is a simple S-shaped tube that allows you to breathe with your head underwater as you move along the surface. You swim or float on the surface of the water and, at times taking a deep breath, surface dive to depths of 15 to 25 feet. With practice you will be able to remain under for 30 seconds or more before returning to the surface for air.

Your safety and pleasure while skin diving are directly related to your level of physical fitness and your swimming ability. A high level of cardiorespiratory endurance is essential if you are to safely enjoy the sport. Without it you cannot dive for long, you will tire easily, and you will not have reserve strength for emergencies. Your legs get the most exercise, but diving and holding your breath can have a conditioning effect on the cardiorespiratory systems if performed regularly.

Just as in most sports, skin diving is best learned from qualified instructors. Swim clubs, YM/YWCAs, and universities usually offer basic instruction. The equipment needed is relatively inexpensive. The fun begins when you have mastered the fundamentals and you have the necessary fitness to dive 20 or 30 feet and stay under for up to a minute.

**Surfing**
The upsurge of interest in surfing in the last 20 years has attracted thousands of people to the seashores. There is no way to express the feeling you can get from a good ride on a big, fast-moving wave. Surfing is

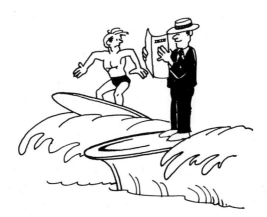

*Surfing*

an individual sport in which one competes with natural forces in total isolation and freedom.

Employing a specially designed board, the surfer rides along beneath the crest of the breaking wave at an angle that depends on the pitch (height) of the wave. The board is controlled by the position of the surfer's body on the board and by the wave itself. Since strong coordination is demanded for maintaining control of the board, you must be in excellent shape to surf. Muscular strength and endurance are mandatory, as is good balance. Paddling the board seaward through and beyond the breaking waves is also extremely demanding. In some seas you may have to paddle continuously for as much as five minutes. During this paddle out, the muscles of the back, chest, shoulders, and arms are taxed greatly, as is the cardiorespiratory system. Dedicated surfers have been known to supplement their surfing activities with leg exercises and vigorous swimming or jogging.

Surfing is not limited to people who can navigate the large-breaking waves. Beginners can find small waves for the first few months until their skills are developed. Instruction is offered by some commercial shops and by fellow surfers. A suitable surfboard can be purchased for under $100, but deluxe models will cost over $250. Commercial shops and resort hotels often rent boards to tourists for a daily fee. For the advanced surfer, there is competition sponsored by national clubs.

## Swimming
Swimming is a universally popular sport. Everyone should learn to swim, if only to be safe when in or near water. But good swimming skills open the door to unlimited recreational possibilities as well.

Once their fear of water is removed, most people experience a feeling of tranquility when floating in water; this buoyancy is a pleasurable and unique feeling. Vigorous swimming, on the other hand, is one of the best forms of physical exercise. Programs of continuous swimming or interval swimming, using such popular strokes as freestyle, backstroke, breaststroke, and sidestroke, have already been described in an earlier chapter. Swimming exerts most of the major muscles of the body, and if you swim fast enough and long enough, you will experience a training effect. Most important, swimming is one of the few sports in this chapter that stresses the cardiorespiratory system substantially. Thus we can quite emphatically say that continuous or interval swimming, when practiced on a regular basis,

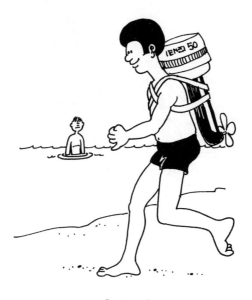

*Swimming*

will contribute to a healthy development and maintenance of your heart, lungs, and muscles.

Water ballet is another form of swimming that has some fitness merit. Swimming clubs and similar organizations often provide programs for performing these specialized stunts and routines in water. Although not as strenuous as endurance or competitive swimming, water ballet exercises involve the entire body and help in maintaining muscle flexibility and tone, and pleasing body contour.

There are countless private clubs, swim schools, recreation centers, colleges, and public schools that offer instruction in swimming for people of all ages and abilities; some of them require membership fees. The cost of qualified instruction in swimming is reasonable when compared with instruction in most other activities. Most of these organizations also sponsor teams for people desiring to compete.

### Tennis
In the United States the popularity of tennis is increasing. With proper instruction you can learn the rudiments of the game in a short time. Once you have reasonably mastered the forehand, backhand, volley, and serve,

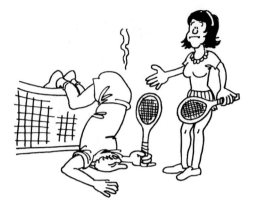

*Tennis*

and some of the footwork needed to get you in position, you are ready for many hours of enjoyable recreation.

Tennis demands coordinated body skill and sufficient strength to control the racquet accurately. The stop-start activity of tennis can be very exhausting at times. Quite often a recreational tennis match can be spoiled by unnecessary fatigue or muscle soreness caused by inadequate physical preparation. But tennis itself will not greatly increase strength, muscular endurance, or cardiorespiratory endurance. These qualities are advantageous for successful play, nevertheless. The tennis player who conditions his cardiorespiratory system with running and tones his muscles with weight training will arm himself with the added factors for success. Many of the world-class tennis players supplement their practice workouts with distance and interval running.

Almost all communities have public tennis courts in parks and other recreation areas. Colleges, country clubs, and private clubs have their own courts, which quite often need to be reserved in advance. New indoor facilities are continually being built, enabling more people to play throughout the year. In many communities, you can find competition no matter what your age, sex, or level of skill. Intramural tournaments are quite common on most college campuses.

Racquets vary in price from $10 to $40 or more. The price reflects the quality of the material used to make the racquet. In addition, you will need good tennis balls, which should be purchased at a reputable sporting goods store. Instruction is recommended if you wish to learn the game and to raise the level of your playing ability. The better you play, the more fun it will be.

### Water Skiing

Water skiing is a popular sport in which over 10 million people participate. The water skier wears one or two skis (five to six feet long) and is towed by a motor boat.

The beginning mechanics are easy to learn, but mastering turns, jumps, and various tricks and stunts takes much skill and practice. Strength, muscular endurance, and flexibility are all important in water skiing. Of particular importance, especially for the highly skilled performer, are posture control and the balance needed to maneuver effectively through more complicated routines.

If you water ski continuously for an extended period of time, your muscle tone and development will undoubtedly be benefited. Crossing wave wakes, jumping, and other riding techniques increase the intensity of the activity. The potential contribution of this sport to cardiorespiratory endurance is somewhat limited, however, since the boat is the main source of propulsion. (On the other hand, the level of your cardiorespiratory fitness determines the overall vigor with which you can water ski. Certainly the

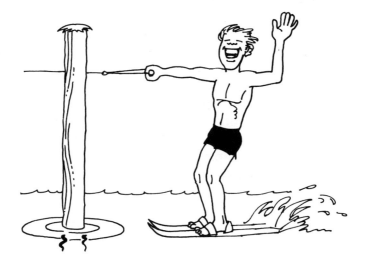

*Water skiing*

physically well-conditioned person will be better able to ski for extended periods.)

When compared to other sporting activities, water skiing is quite costly, though the exact cost depends on how independently you pursue the sport. First, you need access to a lake or large waterway, and a maneuverable boat (15-foot minimum) with a 40- to 75-horsepower motor. The boat and motor together are very expensive, beginning at a minimum of $3000 for new equipment. In addition, you must provide or rent skis, tow ropes, and a life vest, not to mention fuel for the motor. You can't water ski alone, either. A competent driver and qualified observer is required at all times. Furthermore, you need to be at ease in the water and be able to swim well enough to stay afloat for several minutes. If you are fortunate enough to have access to a boat and the necessary equipment, though, water skiing can be an exhilirating experience.

## RATING THE FITNESS POTENTIAL OF LIFETIME SPORTS

As mentioned at the beginning of this chapter, the benefits from sports participation vary from one person to the next. Any attempt to classify activities according to their relative benefits is very limited. Nevertheless, if we accept the philosophy that a healthy functioning of the human organism is benefited by regular muscular exercise, we can then consider the various possibilities for a planned physical activity program that is sufficient for maintaining a healthy well-being. Your limits of physiological fitness development are, of course, dependent on the intensity, duration, and frequency of participation. Throughout the book we have presented some basic activity modes for developing physical fitness on an individualized basis. Applying this knowledge along with your personal desires and goals, the following charts have been devised to assist you in rating the physical potential of various activities. You can make your selection according to your age, skills, and abilities, and the availability of facilities and time. Many of these listed activities are not suitable for daily or four-times-a-week programs. However, they can provide an occasional day or weekend of enjoyable activity to supplement your basic conditioning program. The key is to use this information to set up a regular exercise program to suit your desires and needs.

The following activities provide the *best potential* for developing and maintaining cardiorespiratory fitness.[2]

[2]The participant should be well-skilled in the activity and the intensity of the participation should elicit a vigorous training stimulus on the cardiorespiratory system (75% HR max).

| CONTINUOUS TYPE | INTERMITTENT TYPE |
|---|---|
| Bicycling | Badminton |
| Canoeing | Dancing |
| Cross-country skiing | Gymnastics |
| Jogging and running (distance) | Handball |
| | Ice skating |
| Orienteering | Jog-walk-jog |
| Skin Diving | Racquetball |
| Swimming | Surfing |
| | Tennis |

Below are listed activities with potential for developing and maintaining strength, muscular endurance, and flexibility. The most suitable activities for developing a particular fitness component are indicated by an asterisk.

| STRENGTH | MUSCULAR ENDURANCE | FLEXIBILITY |
|---|---|---|
| Calisthenics | Calisthenics* | Calisthenics* |
| Canoeing | Canoeing* | |
| Cycling | Cycling* | |
| Modern dancing | Modern dancing | Modern dancing* |
| Fencing | | Fencing |
| Gymnastics* | | Gymnastics* |
| | Gymnastics | |
| | Handball* | Handball |
| Hiking | Hiking* | |
| Ice skating | Ice skating | Ice skating |
| | Jogging and running* | |
| Judo* | Judo | Judo* |
| Karate* | Karate* | Karate* |
| | Orienteering* | |
| | Skin diving | Skin diving |
| Skiing (alpine) | Skiing (alpine) | Skiing (alpine) |
| Skiing (cross-country) | Skiing (cross-country)* | Skiing (cross-country) |
| Racquetball | | Racquetball |
| Surfing | Surfing* | Surfing |
| Swimming | Swimming* | Swimming* |
| | Tennis | Tennis |
| Water skiing | Water skiing | Water skiing |
| Weight training* | Weight training* | Weight training |

*Rating the Fitness Potential of Lifetime Sports*    **311**

Here are some activities that can be regulated and performed at a moderate to low intensity level for people with physical limitations.

Bicycling
Calisthenics
Canoeing
Cross-country skiing (touring pace)
Dancing
Hiking
Ice skating
Jog-walk-jog
Swimming
Water skiing

Activities that have limited or no potential for developing muscular endurance and strength, flexibility, or cardiorespiratory endurance are:

Archery
Bowling
Golf

## PRESIDENTIAL SPORTS AWARD PROGRAM

The President's Council on Physical Fitness and Sports has recently inaugurated a *Presidential Sports Award Program.* The program is designed to encourage regular participation in sports. The council has developed qualifying standards for more than 40 participatory sports in cooperation with,

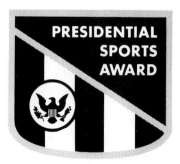

*Presidential sports awards*

and approved by, the appropriate sports governing bodies. Most of the activities presented in this chapter are included in the Presidential Sports Award Program.

The standards are intended to assure regular participation and an investment of enough time and effort to maintain physical fitness. Basically, the standards have been set so that you must invest about three hours a week in your sport over a four-month period to qualify. The award package consists of a lapel pin, a certificate, and an embroidered emblem designating the sport in which the standards were met.

Program information, such as qualifying standards and log books, can be obtained from college intramural departments, YM/YWCAs, and other recreation centers. You can also write directly to

> Presidential Sports Award Program
> P.O. Box 1412
> Annex Station
> Providence, Rhode Island 02904

## FITNESS AND SPORTS: LIFETIME CONCERNS

This chapter has described various sporting activities. You unquestionably should become active in one or more of them. Fitness and sports are lifetime concerns and the sports and leisure activities described can all be engaged in throughout a lifetime. In earlier chapters we have stressed that specific training programs (such as jog-walk-jog, weight training, and circuit training) are the best means for developing all four physical fitness components: strength, muscular endurance, flexibility, and cardiorespiratory endurance. Nevertheless, we recognize the importance of supplementing such programs with other pleasurable sports activities. You should carefully select your sport or sports. They should be enjoyable, suited to your abilities, within your financial means, and convenient to your time and equipment. Some of your favorites may be impossible to pursue on a regular basis, but during vacations, many people travel to the coast for surfing, to the lakes for water skiing, or to the mountains to ski. Don't shy away from unfamiliar sports; too often people limit themselves out of a fear that they will not succeed. Many fine physical education programs around the country now provide instruction in many of the sports reviewed in this chapter. We hope you consider getting involved with one or more of them.

# SUPPLEMENTARY READINGS

ALPINE SKIING

Kidd, Billy and Douglas K. Hall, *Winning Skiing.* Chicago: Henry Regnery, Co., 1975.

Killy, Jean Claude, *Skiing, The Killy Way.* New York: Simon and Schuster, 1971.

Professional Ski Instructors of America, *The Official American Ski Technique.* Cowles Book Company, 1970.

Tucker, Karl and Clayne Jensen, *Skiing.* Dubuque, Iowa: W. C. Brown, 1968.

ARCHERY

Barrett, Jean A., *Archery.* 2nd Edition, Pacific Palisades, California: Goodyear Publishing, 1973.

Campbell, Donald W., *Archery.* Englewood Cliffs, New Jersey: Prentice-Hall, 1971.

BACKPACKING

Elman, Robert, *The Hiker's Bible.* Garden City, New York: Doubleday, 1973.

Manning, Harvey, *Backpacking: One Step At A Time.* Westminister, Maryland, Random House, 1973.

VanLear, Denise, Ed., *The Best About Backpacking.* Totowa, New Jersey: Sierra Club Books, 1974.

CAMPING AND BACKPACKING

Jobson, John, *Complete Book of Practical Camping.* New York: Winchester Press, 1974.

Langer, Richard W., *The Joy of Camping.* New York: Saturday Review Press, 1973.

BADMINTON

Devlin, J. Frank, *Sports Illustrated, Badminton.* Philadelphia: J. G. Lippincott, 1973.

Poole, James, *Badminton.* 2nd Edition, Pacific Palisades: Goodyear Publishing, 1973.

## BICYCLING

DeLong, Fred, *DeLong's Guide to Bicycles and Bicycling.* Radnor, Pennsylvania: Chilton Book, 1974.

Sloane, Eugene A., *The New Complete Book of Bicycling.* New York: Simon and Schuster, 1974.

Thiffault, Mark, *Bicycle Digest.* Chicago: Digest Books, 1973.

## BOWLING

Bellisimo, Lou and Larry Neal, *The Bowlers Manual.* Third Edition, Englewood Cliffs, New Jersey: Prentice-Hall, 1975.

## CANOEING AND KAYAKING

Angier, Bradford and Zack Taylor, *Introduction to Canoeing.* Harrisburg, Pennsylvania: Stackpole Books, 1973.

Bearse, Ray, *The Canoe Camper's Handbook.* New York: Winchester Press, 1974.

Evans, Jay and Robert Anderson, *Kayaking: The New Water Sport for Everyone.* Brattleboro, Vermont: Stephen Greene Press, 1975.

Vaughan, Linda and Richard Stratton, *Canoeing and Sailing.* Dubuque, Iowa: W. C. Brown, 1970.

## CROSS-COUNTRY SKIING

Brunner, Hans and Alois Kälin, *Cross-Country Skiing.* Toronto: McGraw-Hill Ryerson Limited, 1969.

Caldwell, John, *New Cross Country Ski Book.* Fourth Edition, Brattleboro, Vermont: Greene, 1973.

Tokle, Art and Martin Luray, *The Complete Guide to Cross-Country Skiing and Touring.* New York: Holt, Rinehart and Winston, 1973.

## DANCE

Pease, Esther, *Modern Dance.* Dubuque, Iowa: W. C. Brown, 1966.

Penrod, James and Janice Plastine, *The Dancer Prepares, Modern Dance for Beginners.* Palo Alto, Calif.: National Press, 1970.

## DISTANCE RUNNING

Fixx, James F., *The Complete Book of Running.* New York: Random House, 1977.

Henderson, Joe, *Run Gently, Run Long.* Mountain View, California: World Publications, 1974.

Sheehan, George, *Dr. Sheehan on Running.* Mountain View, California: World Publications, 1975.


## FENCING

deBeaumont, Charles, *Fencing.* New York: A. S. Barnes, 1971.

Garret, Maxwell and Mary Heinecke, *Fencing.* Boston: Allyn and Bacon, 1971.


## GOLF

Aultman, Dick, *The Square-To-Square Golf Swing.* New York: Golf Digest, 1970.

Nicklaus, Jack, *Golf My Way.* New York: Simon and Schuster, 1974.

Wiren, Gary, *Golf.* Englewood Cliffs, New Jersey: Prentice-Hall, 1971.


## GYMNASTICS

Carter, Ernestine and Fred Orlofsky, *Beginning Tumbling and Floor Exercise.* Belmont, California: Wadsworth, 1971.

Drury, Blanche, J. and Andrea B. Schmid, *Introduction to Women's Gymnastics.* Palo Alto, Calif.: National Press Books, 1973.

Fogel, Samuel J., *Gymnastics Handbook.* West Nyack, New York: Parker, 1971.


## HANDBALL

Haber, Paul, *Inside Handball.* Chicago: Reilly and Lee Books, 1970.

Nelson, Richard C. and Harlan S. Berger, *Handball.* Englewood Cliffs, New Jersey: Prentice-Hall, 1971.


## ICE SKATING

Proctor, Marion, *Figure Skating.* Dubuque, Iowa: W. C. Brown, 1969.

Ogilvie, Robert S., *Basic Ice Skating Skills.* Philadelphia: J. B. Lippincott, 1968.

Owen, Maribel Vinson, *The Fun of Figure Skating.* New York: Harper and Row, 1960.

## JUDO AND KARATE

Kim, Daeshik, *Judo.* Dubuque, Iowa: W. C. Brown, 1969.

Harrison, Ernest J., *Manual of Karate.* New York: Sterling, 1966.

Kim, Daeshik and Tom Leland, *Karate and Personal Defense.* Dubuque, Iowa: W. C. Brown, 1971.

Tenger, Bruce, *Karate and Judo Exercises: Conditioning for the Oriental Sport Fighting Arts.* Ventura, Calif.: Thor, 1972.

## ORIENTEERING

Disley, John, *Orienteering.* Harrisburg, Pennsylvania: Stackpole Books, 1969.

Kjellstrom, Bjorn, *Be Expert With Map and Compass: The Orienteering Handbook.* Totowa, New Jersey: Scribner's, 1972.

## RACQUETBALL

Keeley, Steve, *The Complete Book of Racquetball.* North Field, Illinois: DB1 Books, 1976.

Spear, Victor, *How to Win at Racquetball.* Rockford, Illinois: Win Publishing, 1974.

Strandemo, Steve, *The Racquetball Book.* New York: Pocket Books, 1977.

## SKIN AND SCUBA DIVING

Council for National Cooperation in Aquatics, *New Science of Skin and Scuba Diving.* New York: Associated Press, 1974.

Tillman, Albert A., *Skin and Scuba Diving.* Dubuque, Iowa: W. C. Brown, 1966.

## SURFING

Dixon, Peter L., *The Complete Book of Surfing.* New York: Coward-McCann, 1965.

Kuhns, Grant W., *On Surfing.* Rutland, Vermont: Charles E. Tuttle, 1963.

Abbot, Rich, *The Science of Surfing.* Newark, New Jersey: International Publications Service, 1974.

Wagenwood, James and Lynn Bailey, *How to Surf.* Riverside, New Jersey: Macmillan, 1968.

## SWIMMING

Armbruster, David A., Robert H. Allen, and Hobert Billingsley, *Swimming and Diving.* 6th Edition, St. Louis: Mosby, 1973.

Collis, Martin and Bill Kirchoff, *Swimming.* Boston: Allyn and Bacon, 1974.

Midtlyng, Joanna, *Swimming.* Philadelphia: W. B. Saunders, 1974.

Sava, Charles, *How to Teach Yourself and Your Family to Swim Well.* New York, Simon and Schuster, 1960.

## TENNIS

Plagenhoef, Stanley, *Fundamentals of Tennis.* Englewood Cliffs, New Jersey: Prentice-Hall, 1970.

Gould, Dick, *Tennis, Anyone?* 2nd Edition, Palo Alto, California: National Press Books, 1971.

King, Billie Jean and Joe Hyams, *Billie Jean King's Secrets of Winning Tennis.* New York: Holt, Rinehart and Winston, 1974.

Pelton, Barry C., *Tennis.* Second Edition, Pacific Palisades: Goodyear Publishing, 1973.

## WATER SKIING

Hester, Ralph, *Instant Water Skiing.* New York: Grosset & Dunlap, 1965.

Tyll, Al, *Water Skiing.* Garden City, New Jersey: Doubleday, 1966.

# epilogue

Since the first edition of this book (1976), various publications have been devoted to the increasing numbers of people exercising. The impression given is that everyone is jogging, cycling, swimming, or playing tennis and racquetball. There are indeed more sport and fitness participants today then ever before, but we wonder how regular their participation is. For example, it has been estimated that there are 103 million swimmers in the United States. Yet, how many actually swim at an intensity and duration that will benefit their cardiorespiratory fitness? How many should we classify as "sunbathers" rather than swimmers? Take racquetball, an excellent sport for all ages. How many of the growing memberships of local clubs actually play on a sufficiently regular basis to improve and maintain a good level of fitness? Having a membership or owning a racquet doesn't guarantee physical fitness. Many of the statistics of the "fitness boom" are supplied by manufacturers eager to promote their equipment. Quite often sports-participant surveys include people who may have played a particular sport only a few times during the year—so anyone with a bicycle hanging in the garage may be listed as a cyclist.

Thus, although there appears to be a national movement toward being more active, we still have a long way to go in informing people about selecting suitable activities for developing and maintaining fitness for a lifetime.

It is encouraging to know there is a greater awareness among people of the need to participate in exercise on a regular basis. In addition, a greater availablity of facilities and chances to participate have improved. For example, the opportunity to test your limits in road races and marathons (26.2 miles) has increased three to fourfold in the last few years. Let's hope this running enthusiasm along with other booms, such as racquetball and tennis, continues to prosper.

In conclusion, we would like to iterate the philosophy that has dominated this book. The quality of your life is determined by the state of your health. Dynamic physical health—one phase of *total* health—is something you cannot buy at the corner drugstore. Instead, it is obtained through vigorous, total-body movement that stimulates the heart, lungs, and muscles substantially on a regular and sustained basis. There is no magical or easy way to get or keep in shape; it takes considerable physical effort. The physically

**320**

fit individual has a definite advantage for enjoyment of meaningful and satisfying living. The decision to be active, to be physically fit, is an individual choice. It involves a process of balance and compromise and it involves priorities. Your health and well-being can be improved and maintained by devoting two or three hours of your time per week to vigorous (not exhaustive) training. You can enjoy all the modern conveniences of transportation and improved technical devices while offsetting this comfortable inactive living style with your personalized fitness program.

An exercise program designed to enlarge your heart's reserve capacities, condition your lungs and blood vessels to function at a greater work load, and achieve overall fitness is necessary. In other words, you exercise to live a quality life, to live at your physiological potential; when you achieve this, you will feel better about yourself, others, and life. Therefore, the aim of this book has been to establish a need for rational and beneficial physical activity to offset the increasing inactivity so characteristic of our daily environment and to provide guidelines for developing a personalized fitness program.

# APPENDIX

# TABLE A.1 T-SCORE: WOMEN. CONVERSION TABLE, RAW SCORES TO T-SCORES

| T-SCORE | GRIP | ONE MIN SIT-UPS | MODIFIED PULL-UPS | VERTICAL JUMP | AGILITY RUN | SQUAT THRUSTS | MILE | 1.5 MILE | STEP TEST |
|---|---|---|---|---|---|---|---|---|---|
| 80 | 45.0 | 45 | 41 | 20.0 | 15.9 | 19-0 | 5:00 | 9:54 | 95 |
| 79 | 44.5 | 44 | 40 | 19.5 | 16.1 | 18-3 | 5:09 | 10:05 | 97 |
| 78 | 44.0 | | | | 16.3 | 18-2 | 5:18 | 10:15 | 100 |
| 77 | 43.5 | 43 | 39 | 19.0 | 16.4 | | 5:27 | 10:26 | 102 |
| 76 | 43.0 | 42 | 38 | | 16.6 | 18-1 | 5:36 | 10:36 | 105 |
| 75 | 42.5 | | | | 16.8 | 18-0 | 5:45 | 10:47 | 107 |
| 74 | 42.0 | 41 | 37 | 18.5 | 17.0 | 17-3 | 5:54 | 10:57 | 109 |
| 73 | 41.5 | 40 | 36 | | 17.2 | 17-2 | 6:03 | 11:08 | 111 |
| 72 | 41.0 | 39 | | 18.0 | 17.3 | | 6:12 | 11:19 | 113 |
| 71 | 40.5 | | 35 | | 17.5 | 17-1 | 6:21 | 11:29 | 116 |
| 70 | 40.0 | 38 | 34 | 17.5 | 17.7 | 17-0 | 6:30 | 11:40 | 118 |
| 69 | 39.5 | 37 | 33 | | 17.9 | 16-3 | 6:39 | 11:51 | 120 |
| 68 | 39.0 | | | 17.0 | 18.1 | 16-2 | 6:48 | 12:01 | 123 |
| 67 | 38.5 | 36 | 32 | | 18.2 | | 6:57 | 12:11 | 125 |
| 66 | 38.0 | 35 | 31 | 16.5 | 18.4 | 16-1 | 7:06 | 12:22 | 127 |
| 65 | 37.5 | | | | 18.6 | 16-0 | 7:15 | 12:33 | 130 |
| 64 | 37.0 | 34 | 30 | | 18.8 | 15-3 | 7:24 | 12:44 | 132 |
| 63 | 36.5 | 33 | 29 | 16.0 | 19.0 | 15-2 | 7:33 | 12:54 | 134 |
| 62 | 36.0 | 32 | | | 19.1 | | 7:42 | 13:05 | 136 |
| 61 | 35.5 | | 28 | 15.5 | 19.3 | 15-1 | 7:51 | 13:15 | 139 |
| 60 | 35.0 | 31 | 27 | | 19.5 | 15-0 | 8:00 | 13:26 | 141 |
| 59 | 34.5 | 30 | 26 | 15.0 | 19.7 | 14-3 | 8:09 | 13:37 | 143 |
| 58 | 34.0 | | | | 19.9 | 14-2 | 8:18 | 13:47 | 146 |
| 57 | 33.5 | 29 | 25 | 14.5 | 20.0 | | 8:27 | 13:58 | 148 |

| T-SCORE | GRIP | ONE MIN SIT-UPS | MODIFIED PULL-UPS | VERTICAL JUMP | AGILITY RUN | SQUAT THRUSTS | MILE | 1.5 MILE | STEP TEST |
|---|---|---|---|---|---|---|---|---|---|
| 56 | 33.0 | 28 | 24 |  | 20.2 | 14-1 | 8:36 | 14:08 | 150 |
| 55 | 32.5 |  |  |  | 20.4 | 14-0 | 8:45 | 14:19 | 153 |
| 54 | 32.0 | 27 | 23 | 14.0 | 20.6 | 13-3 | 8:54 | 14:30 | 155 |
| 53 | 31.5 | 26 | 22 |  | 20.8 | 13-2 | 9:03 | 14:40 | 157 |
| 52 | 31.0 |  |  | 13.5 | 20.9 |  | 9:12 | 14:51 | 159 |
| 51 | 30.5 | 25 | 21 |  | 21.1 | 13-1 | 9:21 | 15:01 | 162 |
| 50 | 30.0 | 24 | 20 | 13.0 | 21.3 | 13-0 | 9:30 | 15:12 | 164 |
| 49 | 29.5 | 23 | 19 |  | 21.5 | 12-3 | 9:39 | 15:23 | 166 |
| 48 | 29.0 |  |  | 12.5 | 21.7 | 12-2 | 9:48 | 15:33 | 169 |
| 47 | 28.5 | 22 | 18 |  | 21.8 |  | 9:57 | 15:44 | 171 |
| 46 | 28.0 | 21 | 17 | 12.0 | 22.0 | 12-1 | 10:06 | 15:54 | 173 |
| 45 | 27.5 |  |  |  | 22.2 | 12-0 | 10:15 | 16:04 | 176 |
| 44 | 27.0 | 20 | 16 |  | 22.4 | 11-3 | 10:24 | 16:15 | 178 |
| 43 | 26.5 | 19 | 15 | 11.5 | 22.6 | 11-2 | 10:33 | 16:26 | 180 |
| 42 | 26.0 |  |  |  | 22.7 |  | 10:42 | 16:36 | 182 |
| 41 | 25.5 | 18 | 14 | 11.0 | 22.9 | 11-1 | 10:51 | 16:47 | 185 |
| 40 | 25.0 | 17 | 13 |  | 23.1 | 11-0 | 11:00 | 16:57 | 187 |
| 39 | 24.5 | 16 | 12 | 10.5 | 23.3 | 10-3 | 11:09 | 17:08 | 189 |
| 38 | 24.0 |  |  |  | 23.5 | 10-2 | 11:18 | 17:19 | 192 |
| 37 | 23.5 | 15 | 11 | 10.0 | 23.6 |  | 11:27 | 17:29 | 194 |
| 36 | 23.0 | 14 | 10 |  | 23.8 | 10-1 | 11:36 | 17:40 | 196 |
| 35 | 22.5 |  |  | 9.5 | 24.0 | 10-0 | 11:46 | 17:50 | 199 |
| 34 | 22.0 | 13 | 9 |  | 24.2 | 9-3 | 11:54 | 18:01 | 201 |
| 33 | 21.5 | 12 | 8 | 9.0 | 24.4 | 9-2 | 12:03 | 18:12 | 203 |

# TABLE A.1   T-SCORE: WOMEN. CONVERSION TABLE, RAW SCORES TO T-SCORES (continued)

| T-SCORE | GRIP | ONE MIN SIT-UPS | MODIFIED PULL-UPS | VERTICAL JUMP | AGILITY RUN | SQUAT THRUSTS | MILE | 1.5 MILE | STEP TEST |
|---|---|---|---|---|---|---|---|---|---|
| 32 | 21.0 |    |    |     | 24.5 |     | 12:12 | 18:22 | 205 |
| 31 | 20.5 | 11 | 7  |     | 24.7 | 9-1 | 12:21 | 18:33 | 208 |
| 30 | 20.0 | 10 | 6  | 8.5 | 24.9 | 9-0 | 12:30 | 18:43 | 210 |
| 29 | 19.5 | 9  | 5  |     | 25.1 | 8-3 | 12:39 | 18:54 | 212 |
| 28 | 19.0 |    |    | 8.0 | 25.3 | 8-2 | 12:48 | 19:05 | 215 |
| 27 | 18.5 | 8  | 4  |     | 25.4 |     | 12:57 | 19:15 | 217 |
| 26 | 18.0 | 7  | 3  | 7.5 | 25.6 | 8-1 | 13:06 | 19:26 | 219 |
| 25 | 17.5 |    |    |     | 25.8 | 8-0 | 13:15 | 19:36 | 222 |
| 24 | 17.0 | 6  | 2  |     | 26.0 | 7-3 | 13:24 | 19:47 | 224 |
| 23 | 16.5 | 5  | 1  | 7.0 | 26.2 | 7-2 | 13:33 | 19:58 | 226 |
| 22 | 16.0 |    | 0  |     | 26.3 |     | 13:42 | 20:08 | 228 |
| 21 | 15.5 | 4  | 0  | 6.5 | 26.5 | 7-1 | 13:51 | 20:19 | 231 |
| 20 | 15.0 | 3  | 0  |     | 26.7 | 7-0 | 14:00 | 20:29 | 233 |

| T-SCORE | GRIP | TWO MIN SIT-UPS | PULL-UPS | DIPS | VERTICAL JUMP | AGILITY RUN | SQUAT THRUSTS | MILE | 2 MILE | STEP TEST |
|---|---|---|---|---|---|---|---|---|---|---|
| 80 | 73 | 91 | 19 | 28 | 27.5 | 15.3 | 23-0 | 4:15 | 10:14 | 97 |
| 79 | 72 | 90 | | | | 15.4 | 22-3 | 4:20 | 10:23 | 99 |
| 78 | 71.5 | 88 | | 27 | 27.0 | | 22-2 | 4:24 | 10:32 | 101 |
| 77 | 71 | 87 | 18 | | | 15.5 | | 4:29 | 10:41 | 103 |
| 76 | 70 | 86 | | 26 | | 15.6 | 22-1 | 4:33 | 10:50 | 105 |
| 75 | 69.5 | 85 | 17 | | 26.5 | 15.7 | 22-0 | 4:38 | 10:59 | 107 |
| 74 | 69 | 84 | | 25 | | 15.8 | 21-3 | 4:42 | 11:08 | 109 |
| 73 | 68 | 83 | | | 26.0 | | 21-2 | 4:47 | 11:17 | 111 |
| 72 | 67 | 81 | 16 | 24 | | 15.9 | | 4:51 | 11:26 | 113 |
| 71 | 66.5 | 80 | | | | 16.0 | 21-1 | 4:56 | 11:35 | 115 |
| 70 | 65.5 | 79 | 15 | 23 | 25.5 | 16.1 | 21-0 | 5:00 | 11:44 | 117 |
| 69 | 65 | 78 | | | | 16.2 | 20-3 | 5:05 | 11:53 | 119 |
| 68 | 64 | 77 | | 22 | 25.0 | | 20-2 | 5:09 | 12:02 | 121 |
| 67 | 63.5 | 76 | 14 | | | 16.3 | | 5:14 | 12:11 | 123 |
| 66 | 63 | 74 | | 21 | | 16.4 | 20-1 | 5:18 | 12:20 | 125 |
| 65 | 62 | 73 | 13 | | 24.5 | 16.5 | 20-0 | 5:23 | 12:29 | 127 |
| 64 | 61 | 72 | | 20 | | 16.6 | 19-3 | 5:27 | 12:38 | 129 |
| 63 | 60.5 | 71 | | | 24.0 | | 19-2 | 5:32 | 12:47 | 131 |
| 62 | 60 | 70 | 12 | 19 | | 16.7 | 19-1 | 5:36 | 12:56 | 133 |
| 61 | 59 | 69 | | | | 16.8 | | 5:41 | 13:05 | 135 |
| 60 | 58.5 | 67 | 11 | 18 | 23.5 | 16.9 | 19-0 | 5:45 | 13:14 | 137 |
| 59 | 58 | 66 | | | | 17.0 | 18-3 | 5:50 | 13:23 | 139 |
| 58 | 57 | 65 | | 17 | 23.0 | | 18-2 | 5:54 | 13:32 | 141 |
| 57 | 56 | 64 | 10 | | | 17.1 | | 5:59 | 13:41 | 143 |

## TABLE A.2  T-SCORE: MEN. CONVERSION TABLE, RAW SCORES TO T-SCORES (continued)

| T-SCORE | GRIP | TWO MIN SIT-UPS | PULL-UPS | DIPS | VERTICAL JUMP | AGILITY RUN | SQUAT THRUSTS | MILE | 2 MILE | STEP TEST |
|---|---|---|---|---|---|---|---|---|---|---|
| 56 | 55.5 | 63 |   | 16 |   |   | 18-1 | 6:03 | 13:50 | 145 |
| 55 | 55 | 62 | 9 |   | 22.5 | 17.2 | 18-0 | 6:08 | 13:59 | 147 |
| 54 | 54 | 60 |   | 15 |   | 17.3 | 17-3 | 6:12 | 14:08 | 149 |
| 53 | 53 | 59 | 8 |   | 22.0 | 17.4 | 17-2 | 6:17 | 14:17 | 151 |
| 52 | 52.5 | 58 |   | 14 |   |   |   | 6:21 | 14:28 | 153 |
| 51 | 52 | 57 | 7 |   |   | 17.5 | 17-1 | 6:26 | 14:37 | 155 |
| 50 | 51 | 56 |   | 13 | 21.5 | 17.6 | 17-0 | 6:30 | 14:46 | 157 |
| 49 | 50.5 | 55 |   |   |   | 17.7 | 16-3 | 6:35 | 14:55 | 159 |
| 48 | 50 | 54 |   | 11 | 21.0 | 17.8 | 16-2 | 6:39 | 15:04 | 161 |
| 47 | 49 | 52 | 6 |   |   |   |   | 6:44 | 15:13 | 163 |
| 46 | 48 | 51 |   | 10 |   | 17.9 | 16-1 | 6:48 | 15:22 | 165 |
| 45 | 47.5 | 50 | 5 |   | 20.5 | 18.0 | 16-0 | 6:53 | 15:31 | 167 |
| 44 | 47 | 49 |   | 9 |   | 18.1 | 15-3 | 6:57 | 15:40 | 169 |
| 43 | 46 | 48 |   |   | 20.0 | 18.2 | 15-2 | 7:02 | 15:49 | 171 |
| 42 | 45 | 46 | 4 | 8 |   |   |   | 7:06 | 15:58 | 173 |
| 41 | 44.5 | 45 |   |   |   | 18.3 | 15-1 | 7:11 | 16:07 | 175 |
| 40 | 44 | 44 | 3 | 7 | 19.5 | 18.4 | 15-0 | 7:15 | 16:16 | 177 |
| 39 | 43 | 43 |   |   |   | 18.5 | 14-3 | 7:20 | 16:25 | 179 |
| 38 | 42 | 42 |   | 6 | 19.0 | 18.6 | 14-2 | 7:24 | 16:34 | 181 |
| 37 | 41.5 | 41 | 2 |   |   |   |   | 7:29 | 16:43 | 183 |
| 36 | 41 | 39 |   | 5 |   | 18.7 | 14-1 | 7:33 | 16:52 | 185 |
| 35 | 40 | 38 | 1 |   | 18.5 | 18.8 | 14-0 | 7:38 | 17:01 | 187 |
| 34 | 39.5 | 37 |   | 4 |   | 18.9 | 13-3 | 7:42 | 17:10 | 189 |
| 33 | 38.5 | 36 |   |   | 18.0 | 19.0 | 13-2 | 7:47 | 17:19 | 191 |

# TABLE A.2  T-SCORE: MEN. CONVERSION TABLE, RAW SCORES TO T-SCORES (continued)

| T-SCORE | GRIP | TWO MIN SIT-UPS | PULL-UPS | DIPS | VERTICAL JUMP | AGILITY RUN | SQUAT THRUSTS | MILE | 2 MILE | STEP TEST |
|---|---|---|---|---|---|---|---|---|---|---|
| 32 | 38 | 35 | 0 | 3 | | 19.1 | | 7:51 | 17:28 | 193 |
| 31 | 37 | 33 | | | | 19.2 | 13-1 | 7:56 | 17:37 | 195 |
| 30 | 36.5 | 32 | | 2 | 17.5 | 19.3 | 13-0 | 8:00 | 17:46 | 197 |
| 29 | 36 | 31 | | | | 19.4 | 12-3 | 8:05 | 17:55 | 199 |
| 28 | 35 | 30 | | 1 | 17.0 | | 12-2 | 8:09 | 18:04 | 201 |
| 27 | 34 | 29 | | | | 19.5 | | 8:14 | 18:13 | 203 |
| 26 | 33.5 | 28 | | 0 | | 19.6 | 12-1 | 8:18 | 18:22 | 205 |
| 25 | 33 | 26 | | | 16.5 | 19.7 | 12-0 | 8:23 | 18:31 | 207 |
| 24 | 32 | 25 | | | | 19.8 | 11-3 | 8:27 | 18:40 | 209 |
| 23 | 31.5 | | | | 16.0 | | 11-2 | 8:32 | 18:49 | 211 |
| 22 | 30.5 | | | | | 19.9 | | 8:36 | 18:58 | 213 |
| 21 | 30 | | | | | 20.0 | 11-1 | 8:41 | 19:07 | 215 |
| 20 | 29 | | | | 15.5 | 20.1 | 11-0 | 8:45 | 19:16 | 217 |

# BODY COMPOSITION CHART

Date _____

Name _____ Age _____ Sex _____

Body weight _____ lbs          (_____ kg)

Skinfold measurements (mm)

      Women:  Tricep _____          Suprailiac _____

      Men:  Subscapular _____          Thigh _____

Percentage of body fat _____(estimated from the Sloan Formulas)

Desired Weight:  Computation                              (1 lb = 0.45 kg)

  1. Fat Weight = Weight × % Fat

$$\text{Fat Weight} = \text{Weight} \times \frac{\% \text{ Fat}}{100}$$

    = _____ × _____ = _____ lb    (_____ kg)

               100

  2. Fatfree Weight = Weight–Fat Weight

    = _____ − _____ = _____ lb    (_____ kg)

  3. Desired Weight (Choose one)

      At 20% fat = fatfree weight/0.80 _____ lb    (_____ kg)

      At 18% fat = fatfree weight/0.82 _____ lb    (_____ kg)

      At 16% fat = fatfree weight/0.84 _____ lb    (_____ kg)

      At 14% fat = fatfree weight/0.86 _____ lb    (_____ kg)

      At 12% fat = fatfree weight/0.88 _____ lb    (_____ kg)

# PHYSICAL FITNESS PROFILE

Date _____

Instructor _____

Name _____ Age _____ Sex _____

     (last)          (first)

Body weight _____ lb  (_____ kg)   Percent body fat _____

Summary of physical fitness evaluation:

| | Raw Score | | T-Scores* | Rating† |
|---|---|---|---|---|
| **Muscular strength and endurance** | | | | |
| Grip strength (dominant) | _____ | kg. | _____ | _____ |
| Sit-ups (bent knees) | _____ | no. | _____ | _____ |
| Pull-ups | _____ | no. | _____ | _____ |
| Dips | _____ | no. | _____ | _____ |
| **Motor performance** | | | | |
| Agility run | _____ | sec. | _____ | _____ |
| Vertical jump | _____ | in. | _____ | _____ |
| Squat thrusts | _____ | no. | _____ | _____ |
| **Cardiorespiratory‡‡ endurance** | | | | |
| 1-Mile run | _____ | min. | _____ | _____ |
| 1.5 Mile run | _____ | min. | _____ | _____ |
| 2-Mile run | _____ | min. | _____ | _____ |
| 12-Minute run | _____ | distance | _____ | _____ |
| Step test (recovery index) | _____ | beats | _____ | _____ |

*T-Scores are derived by converting the raw measurements (i.e. inches, seconds, number, etc.) of each distribution to a common scale of comparable units. Refer to the Appendix for the conversion table, Tables A.1 or A.2. Raw scores to T-Scores.

‡To rate each test according to classifiction tables, Tables 3.1 to 3.8.

‡‡Select only one running test plus the recovery index.

To compute your average T-score for all tests taken, sum the scores and divide by the number of tests completed.

_____

(sum of all tests) ÷ (number of tests) = (average T-score)

             A T-score above 55 is considered *good*.

# PHYSICAL FITNESS PROFILE

Date _____

Instructor _____

Name _____ Age _____ Sex _____
    (last)      (first)

Body weight _____ lb   (_____ kg)  Percent body fat _____

|  | Raw Score | T-score |
|---|---|---|
| Muscular strength and endurance | | |
| Sit-ups (bent knee) | _____ no. | _____ |
| Pull-ups | _____ no. | _____ |
| Motor performance | | |
| Agility run | _____ sec | _____ |
| Vertical jump | _____ in. | _____ |
| Cardiorespiratory endurance | | |
| Distance run (perform one) | | |

1-Mile _____; 1.5-Mile _____; 2-Mile _____     _____
  (min:sec)      (min:sec)      (min:sec)

To compute your average T-score sum the T-scores for the 5 tests or 3 tests (sit-ups, pull-ups, and distance run) and divide by 5 or 3, respectively.

_____

Sum of 5 tests ÷ 5 = Average T-score

_____

Sum of 3 tests ÷ 3 = Average T-score

Your T-score for the 5 ITEM is _____; Rating _____.

Your T-score for the 3 ITEM is _____; Rating _____.

# GLOSSARY

ADENOSINE TRIPHOSPHATE (ATP): A high energy substance found in all cells from which the body gets its energy.

AEROBIC CAPACITY: A functional measure of physical fitness based on the measurement of maximal oxygen uptake. Generally synonymous with the terms maximal oxygen uptake and cardiorespiratory endurance.

ALVEOLI: Tiny air sacs in the lungs where rapid exchange of the respiratory gases takes place with the blood in the adjacent capillaries.

AMINO ACIDS: The end product of the breakdown of protein.

ANAEROBIC: "Without oxygen"; the output of energy for muscular contraction when the oxygen supply is insufficient.

ARTERIOSCLEROSIS: The advanced stage of atherosclerosis when the arteries become hardened.

ARTERY: An elastic vessel that transports blood away from the heart.

ATHEROSCLEROSIS: The deposits and build-up of fatty substances on the inner walls of the arteries.

ATRIUM: One of the upper chambers of the heart. The right atrium receives "used" blood from the systems of the body and the left atrium receives oxygenated blood from the lungs.

BASAL METABOLIC RATE (BMR): The minimal rate of energy required to maintain the life processes of the body during a resting state following at least twelve hours of not eating.

333

BLOOD PRESSURE: The force that blood exerts against the walls of the blood vessels and that makes the blood flow through the circulatory system.

BLOOD SUGAR: The glucose concentrations in the blood. This term should not be confused with refined sugar. See SUGAR.

BODY DENSITY: The compactness of the body, equal to the body weight divided by the body volume.

BRONCHIOLES: Smaller branches of each bronchus in the lungs.

BRONCHUS: One of the two air tubes that branch off from the trachea to each lung.

CALORIE: A unit of measure for the rate of heat or energy production in the body.

CAPILLARIES: The smallest vessels in the circulatory system where all exchanges of nutrients and respiratory gases take place between the blood and tissues.

CARBOHYDRATES: A food substance that is the primary energy food for vigorous muscular activity. Includes various sugars and starches and is found in the body in the form of glucose and glycogen.

CARBON DIOXIDE: The waste gas given off during the breakdown of foodstuffs in the cell and transported in the blood to the lungs and exhaled.

CARDIAC: Relating to the heart, such as cardiac output, cardiac muscle, and so on.

CARDIAC OUTPUT: The amount of blood pumped by the heart per minute. The product of stroke volume times the heart rate.

CARDIORESPIRATORY: Joint functioning of the circulatory system (heart and blood vessels) and the respiratory system (the lungs, air passages).

CARDIORESPIRATORY ENDURANCE: The capacity of your heart, blood vessels, and lungs to function efficiently during vigorous, sustained activity such as jogging, swimming, and cycling. See AEROBIC CAPACITY.

CHOLESTEROL: A waxy, fatty-like substance that serves an important role as a building block for formation of essential compounds vital to body functions. It is produced in the body and also obtained by eating foods of animal origin. Elevated levels in the blood have been associated with an increased risk of heart and blood vessel disease.

CIRCUIT TRAINING: A routine of selected exercises or activities performed in sequence at individual stations, as rapidly as possible.

CONDITIONING BOUT: The main exercise portion of a workout with a training intensity level at a heart rate approximating 75 percent of the difference between resting and maximal heart rates.

CONTINUOUS TRAINING: Sustaining a constant tempo of exercise for a period of time. In beginning programs, bouts of brisk walking are generally alternated with short bouts of exercise.

COOL-DOWN: The tapering off period after completion of the main conditioning bout, with activities such as slow jogging, walking, and stretching the major muscle groups.

CORONARY ARTERIES: The arteries that supply blood and nourishment to the heart muscle.

CORONARY HEART DISEASE: The impairment of the arteries of the heart (coronaries) from a build-up of cholesterol and associated fatty substances on the inner portion of the artery wall. See ATHEROSCLEROSIS.

CREATINE PHOSPHATE (CP): An energy-rich compound that plays a key role in providing energy for instant muscle contraction.

DIABETES: A chronic disorder of glucose (sugar) metabolism due to a disturbance of the normal insulin mechanism. See INSULIN.

DIASTOLIC PRESSURE: The lowest force exerted by the arterial blood flow against the walls of the vessels.

DISTANCE REPEATS: The repeated bouts of alternate jogging and walking using specified distances as the determinant of the work load.

DURATION: The term used in prescribing exercise that refers to the time length of training sessions. For example, thirty minutes at an intensity of 75% HR max is the recommended duration for developing and maintaining physical fitness.

ELECTROCARDIOGRAPHY (ECG): The recording of the electrical activity (nervous energy) of the heart.

ENDURANCE: The ability to sustain an activity and resist fatigue. See MUSCULAR ENDURANCE and CARDIORESPIRATORY ENDURANCE.

ENZYMES: An organic substance that speeds up the chemical reactions within the body.

ERGOMETER: A stationary exercise bicycle that can be adjusted to provide an accurate measurement of the work performed.

ESOPHAGUS: The passageway for food from the throat to the stomach.

EXERCISE PRESCRIPTION: Individualizing the exercise workout based on intensity, duration, frequency, and mode of exercise.

FAST TWITCH MUSCLE FIBER: A type of muscle fiber with "fast" contractile characteristics that has a low capacity to use oxygen. These fibers are the first to be used in short sudden burst of activities. See SLOW TWITCH MUSCLE FIBER.

FAT: A food substance used as a source of energy in the body and capable of being stored.

FAT-FREE WEIGHT: Your body weight free of fat (often referred to as lean body weight).

FAT WEIGHT: The absolute amount of body fat.

FATTY ACID: The end product of the breakdown of fats.

FIELD TESTS: Physical fitness tests performed outside the controlled environment of the laboratory (e.g., two-mile run, sit-ups).

FLEXIBILITY: The range of movement of a specific joint and its corresponding muscle groups.

FREQUENCY: The term that refers to the number of workouts needed to reach a training effect in conjunction with the intensity and duration factors recommended.

GLUCOSE: The end product of carbohydrate that is transported in the blood (blood sugar) and metabolized in the cell.

GLYCOGEN: The form in which carbohydrates are stored in the muscles and liver.

GRAM: A unit of mass and weight in the metric system. An ounce equals 28.3 grams, whereas 1000 grams equals one kilogram or 2.2 pounds.

HEART: A powerful muscular pump responsible for blood circulation.

HEART RATE: The number of times the heart beats per minute. In most cases the number of heart beats each minute is equal to the number of pulse beats per minute.

HEMOGLOBIN: The iron-containing protein in the red blood cell that combines readily with carbon dioxide and oxygen and acts as a carrier of these gases throughout the circulatory system.

HYPERTENSION: A higher than normal blood pressure, usually defined as any systolic pressure above 140 mmHg and a diastolic pressure in excess of 90 mmHg.

HYPERTROPHY: The term used to describe the increase in size or mass of a cell, tissue, or organ (e.g., increase in muscle fiber size resulting from strength training).

INSULIN: A hormone that controls the rate of glucose entry into the cell.

INTENSITY: The physiological stress on the body during exercise. Your level of intensity can be readily determined by measuring your pulse rate (heart rate) immediately following an exercise bout.

INTERVAL TRAINING: Successive bouts of exercise at near-maximal intensity, alternated with lighter periods of rest or exercise such as brisk walking.

ISOKINETIC CONTRACTION: A muscle contraction at a constant speed with the muscle generating force against a variable resistance.

ISOMETRIC CONTRACTION: A muscle contraction with the muscle generating force without allowing significant shortening of the muscle (e.g., pushing against a wall).

ISOTONIC CONTRACTION: A muscle contraction with the muscle generating force against a constant resistance with a shortening of the muscle (e.g., curling a barbell).

KILOGRAM: Metric measure of weight; 2.2 pounds equals one kilogram or 1000 grams.

LACTIC ACID: The end product of anaerobic metabolism.

LEAN BODY WEIGHT: The body weight minus the percent of body weight that is stored fat.

LIGAMENT: The connective tissue that binds bones together.

LIPID: A fat, or fat-like substance such as fatty acids, triglycerides and cholesterol.

LIPOPROTEIN: A type of protein that carries cholesterol and triglycerides in the bloodstream.

LITER: Basic metric unit of capacity, equal to 1.06 quarts or 1000 milliliters.

LOAD: The poundage used for a particular weight training exercise.

LUNGS: Located within the rib cage, these two organs regulate the exchange of air between the blood and external environment.

MET: Represents the rate of energy expended at rest; used to rate activities in multiples above rest.

MAXIMAL HEART RATE: The highest attainable heart rate for an individual.

MAXIMAL OXYGEN UPTAKE: The largest amount of oxygen that can be consumed per minute. It is the best physiological index of cardiorespiratory endurance. Often referred to as maximal aerobic capacity, maximal oxygen intake, or maximal oxygen consumption.

MEAN: Commonly understood as the arithmetic average (computed by dividing the sum of all scores by the number of scores).

MENSTRUATION: The periodic cycle in the uterus of the female associated with preparation of the uterus to receive a fertilized egg.

METABOLISM: All the chemical processes of the body that make it possible for the cells to function.

MINERALS: A group of 22 metallic elements vital to proper cell functioning; for example, minerals are part of enzymes, hormones, and vitamins.

MOTOR SKILL: The ability of muscles to function harmoniously and efficiently, resulting in smooth, coordinated muscular movement. A reflection of general athletic skill.

MUSCLE FIBER: A structural unit of muscle. Often referred to as muscle cell.

MUSCULAR ENDURANCE: The capacity of a muscle to exert a force repeatedly or to hold a fixed or static contraction over a period of time.

MYOCARDIAL INFARCTION: Heart attack or death of the heart muscle (myocardium) due to lack of oxygen.

MYOCARDIUM: Heart muscle.

NORM: A standard of achievement represented by the average achievement of a large group.

NUTRIENT: The basic substances of the body that are provided by the eating of foods.

NUTRITION: The study of food and how the body uses it.

OBESITY: An excessive amount of body fat or the state of being too fat.

OVERLOAD PRINCIPLE: The physiological fact that a muscle subjected to a greater-than-normal load will increase in size and strength.

OXIDATIVE: The breakdown of foodstuffs with oxygen to produce energy for reforming ATP. Krebs cycle is another name for this process.

OXYGEN: A colorless, odorless, tasteless, gaseous chemical element that occurs free in the atmospheric air, forming one-fifth of its volume. It is the essential respiratory gas for life processes in the cell.

OXYGENATED: To mix or combine with oxygen, such as the combining of oxygen with the red blood cells in the lungs.

OXYGEN UPTAKE: The amount of energy the body uses; easily converted to Calories.

PLASMA: The fluid part of the blood. See SERUM.

POWER: The rate at which force can be produced or the product of force and velocity; sometimes referred to as the explosive ability to apply force.

PROTEIN: A food substance that provides the basic structural properties of the cells; also the source for enzymes and hormones in the body.

RECOVERY INDEX: The sum of three 30-second heart rate recovery counts after the step test.

RED BLOOD CELLS: The cells of blood that transport hemoglobin, which in turn carries oxygen from the lungs to the tissues.

RELATIVE BODY FAT: The proportion of fat tissue in your body, often expressed as a percentage of body weight. (Percent body fat)

REPETITIONS: The number of consecutive contractions performed during each weight training exercise. See SETS.

REPETITIONS MAXIMUM (RM): The maximum load that can be lifted a given number of times for a particular weight training exercise (e.g., 6 RM is the maximum weight that can be performed 6 times).

RESPIRATION: The process of gas exchange in the lungs and cells of the body.

SATURATED FATS: A food source found in meat, milk, cheese, and butter. This type of fat does not melt at room temperature.

SERUM: The fluid part of the blood after clotting.

SET: The number of bouts performed for each weight training exercise (e.g., 3 sets of 6 reps). See REPETITIONS.

SKINFOLD CALIPER: An instrument used to measure selected thickness of fat folds that have been pinched up on the body.

SLOW TWITCH MUSCLE FIBER: A type of muscle fiber with "slow" contractile characteristics that has a high capacity to use oxygen. These fibers are used primarily during endurance activities such as jogging, swimming, and cycling. See FAST TWITCH MUSCLE FIBER.

STANDARD DEVIATION: A measure of variability that indicates the scatter and spread of approximately two-thirds of a distribution of scores around a mean (see MEAN and NORM).

STEP-TEST: A testing procedure for assessing the heart rate recovery after stepping on and off a bench for a three-minute time period at a predetermined cadence.

STRENGTH: The capacity of a muscle to exert a force against a resistance.

STROKE VOLUME: The volume of blood ejected from the left ventricle during one heart beat.

SUGAR: A term often misused; in this book it refers to refined sugar or table sugar. The scientific name for sugar is sucrose. See BLOOD SUGAR.

SYSTOLIC PRESSURE: The greatest force exerted by the arterial blood flow against the walls of the vessels.

TENDON: An extension of muscle tissue that attaches to the bone.

T-SCORE: A score that enables you to interpret and compare raw scores from various fitness tests. It provides a simple way to describe the deviation of a test result from the average score for the particualr test. See MEAN, STANDARD DEVIATION, and NORM.

TIMED REPEATS: The repeated bouts of alternate jogging and walking using time as the determinant of the work load.

TRACHEA: The windpipe through which air passes to the lungs from the throat.

TRAINING EFFECT: The term used to describe the many physiological changes that result from participation in vigorous, muscular fitness activities.

TRAINING HEART RATE: A heart beat rate (or pulse rate) per minute during exercise that will produce significant cardiorespiratory benefits.

TREADMILL: A testing device consisting of a motor-driven conveyor belt constructed so that the speed and angle of incline can be regulated to produce varying workloads.

TRIGLYCERIDES: Fat particles that are stored in the body. They provide the main means for fat to be transported in the blood. Recent evidence has revealed an association with atherosclerosis. See CHOLES-TEROL.

TYPE A BEHAVIOR: The term used to describe people who exhibit an excessive competitive drive and time urgency. This behavior tends to predispose people to heart disease.

UNSATURATED FATS: A liquid type of fat found in peanut oil and olive oil.

VEIN: A vessel that carries blood back to the heart.

VENTILATION: The movement of volumes of air into and out of the lungs.

VENTRICLE: The chamber of the heart that pumps blood to the lungs (right ventricle) or to all the systems of the body (left ventricle).

VITAMINS: Organic substances that perform vital functions within the cells.

WARM-UP: The exercise portion of your workout that is geared to preparing your body for a more vigorous exercise bout. Generally, walking, stretching major muscle groups, and exercises that stimulate the heart, lungs, and muscles moderately and progressively are engaged in during warm-up periods.

WHITE BLOOD CELLS: The blood cells that provide a rapid and potent defense against infectious agents present in the body.

# INDEX

Activity selection, 99-100, 104-105. *See also*
  Sports; Workouts
Adenosine triphosphate, 32-33
Aerobic capacity, 28-32, 35
  defined, 28-29, 211, 212
  field tests for, 32, 66-69
  measurement of, 28-29
  relationship with anaerobic, 32-33, 211-213
  values, for athletes, 29-30
    college-aged students, 30
    middle-aged adults, 30
  *see also* Cardiorespiratory endurance and
    fitness; Maximal oxygen uptake
Age, decline of fitness and, 9, 31
  designing personal program and, 101
  energy needs and, 230
  heart disease risk and, 257, 259
  maximal oxygen uptake and, 30
Agility run, 62, 215
Alpine skiing, 278
American Alliance for Health, Physical Education
  and Recreation, 6
American Heart Association, 9, 257, 259, 261,
  265, 269
American Medical Association, 269
Amino acids, 223
Anaerobic, defined, 32, 212
  relationship with aerobic, 33, 211-212
  training, 207
Archery, 280
Arm circles, 120-121, 148
Arm curls, 195
Arm and leg lifter, 131, 148, 158
Arteriosclerosis, 258
Astrand, P.O., 269
Atherosclerosis, 258
Athletes, maximal oxygen uptake values, 29-30
Athletic ability, 13, 61. *See also* Evaluation; Motor
  skill performance
Athletics, traditional approach, 6

Attitudes toward exercise, 5-6
  formation of, 6


Backpacking and camping, 281
Back pain, *see* Low back pain
Badminton, 283
Balance, 13
Balke, Bruno, 67-68
Basal metabolic rate, 230, 235
Behavior, Type-A, 265-266
Bench press, 197
Bent-over rowing, 200
Berger, Richard, 193
Bicycle, Ergometer test, 73-75
  stationary bike training, 178-181
  training with, 170-173, 210
Bicycling, 104-105, 170-173, 284
Blood, 22
  hemoglobin, 22, 24, 40
  red blood cells, 22
Blood pressure, 35, 260
  hypertension, 260
Body build, desired girths, 83-84
  desired weight, 84
  development of, 117-120
  evaluation of, 83-84, 238-240
Body composition, chart, 330
  exercise benefits and, 36
Body fat, calculations, 79-81
  estimation of, 238-240
  evaluation, 77-82
  height-weight tables, discussion of, 238
  measurement procedures, 78
  mirror test, 240
  nomograms, 81-82
  norms, 82, 239-240
  skinfold caliper, use of, 78, 239-240
  *see also* Obesity, Weight control; *and* Weight
    reduction

Body weight, determining desirable weight, 85,
    250-251
  height-weight tables, discussion of, 238
  see also Body fat; Obesity; Weight control; and
    Weight reduction
Bowling, 285

Calf stretcher (achilles), 136, 148
Calisthenics, 117-154
  for runners, 149
  see also Exercises, basic conditioning
Caloric cost, calculations of, 230, 235-236,
    241-242
  daily requirements, 230, 235
    of jogging, 243
  measurement of, 241
  METS and, 242-244, 246
  oxygen equivalency, 242
    of selected activities, 243-246
    of sports, 246
  see also Energy cost
Calories, caloric cost of activities, 243-246
  defined, 230
  energy equivalent, 242
  food values (charts), 230-235
  weight loss and, 249-251
Calorimetry, defined, 241
Camaraderie, 109, 171
Camping, 281
Canoeing, 183-184, 286
Carbohydrates, 223-224, 228, 229
Cardiac output, 28
Cardiac rehabilitation, 269
Cardiac risk game, 267-268
Cardiorespiratory endurance and fitness, benefits
    of, 34-35
  conditioning for, 162-187, 206-217
  defined, 13-14
  designing program for, 101-104
  development of, 93-100
  evaluation of, 65-77
  field tests for, 66-72
  golf and, 99, 292
  need for, 10
  swimming and, 174-176
  weight training and, 192, 195
Cardiovascular system, 22
Cell, 21, 22
Childbirth, 41
Cholesterol, 35, 225
  heart disease and, 258, 260-262
Circuit training, 213-216

  definition and explanation, 207, 213-216
Classification tables, cardiorespiratory endurance,
    72, 73
  1.5 mile run for females, 69
  2.0 mile run for males, 69
  flexibility, 58-60
  interpretation of, 50-51
  motor skill performance, 65
  muscular strength and endurance, 57-58
  rating your fitness, 50-51
  T-scores, explanation, 50-51
  see also Evaluation
Clothing, in cold weather, 106-107
  for exercising, 106
  in hot weather, 106, 248-249
  for weight training, 193
  for women, bra, 106-107
  see also Chapter 11
Conditioning, advanced, 206-217
  principles of, 93-101
  three-segment workout, 102-104
  see also Exercises
Continuous training, 163, 207, 210-213, 310-311
Cool-down, 103
Cooper, Ken, 38, 68
Coronary arteries, 24, 258
Coronary heart disease, 163, 257. See also Heart
    disease
Costill, David, 263
Counsilman, James, 202
Creatine phosphate, 33
Cross-country skiing, 184-185, 288
Cureton, Thomas K., 7
Curl-up, half, 145, 158

Dance, 289
Death, heart disease statistics, 257, 259
  heat stroke, 249
  myocardial infarction, 258
Dehydration, 248-249
Diabetes, 263
Diet, 9-10
  basics for nutritional diet, 228-229
  caloric value of foods, 231-235
  crash diets, 240
  exercise and, 118, 240-246, 249-251
  heart disease and, 260-262
  high fat, 260-262
  lifetime philosophy, 251
  national goals, 227-228
  plan for losing weight, 249-251
  see also Obesity; Weight control

Dips, 55
Distance running, 290

Effects and benefits of excercise, aging 31,
        271-272
    body fat, 36
    cardiorespiratory, 13-14, 34-35
    psychological, 16-17, 36-38
Emergencies, fitness and, 9
Emotions, heart disease and, 265
Emphysema, 264
Endurance, see Cardiorespiratory endurance and
        fitness; Muscular endurance
Energy cost, activities, 243, 246
    calculation of, 242-245
    calories, 230, 235-236
    daily, 230, 235-236
    METS, 242-244
    oxygen use and, 241-242
    table, for daily expenditures, 236
        for jogging, 243
        for selected activities, 246
    see also Caloric cost
Enjoyment, 16-17, 101
Evaluation, body composition chart, 230
    body fat and build, 77-85
    cardiorespiratory endurance, 28, 32, 66-77
    conversion charts, 324-329
    flexibility, 58-60
    heart disease risk, 267-268
    medical exam, 48, 93
    motor skill, 61-65
    muscular strength and endurance, 51-57
    profile charts, 87, 88, 331, 332
    rating of sports for fitness development, 310-312
    T-scores, 50-51
    see also Classification tables
Exercise, appetite and, 246
    benefits, of, 33-38
    camaraderie, 109
    in cold weather, 105, 107
    duration, 98, 100
    effects from lack of, 7-9
    energy expenditure, 241
    frequency, 98-99, 100
    heart and, 25
    heart response to exercise, 26-27
    in hot humid weather, 105-106, 248-249
    intensity and, 93-98, 100-101, 164-165
    negative approach, 5
    positive approach, 6-7, 271
    precautions, 48, 107, 109-110, 177-178

prescription factors for, 93-104
preventive measure for heart disease, 8, 269-272
    in rain, 105
    reasons for, 6, 10, 14-17
    spot reducing, 247
    three segment workout, 102-104, 172-173
    warm-up, 102
    weight control, 240-246
    when and where to workout, 105-106
    women and, 39-41, 119
    see also Exercises
Exercises, basic conditioning, 117-154
    arm and leg lifter, 131, 148, 158
    arm circles, 120-121, 148
    back-over, 138
    calf stretcher (achilles), 136, 137, 148
    cat-stretch, 154
    chest and shoulder developer, 151
    chest developer, 149-150
    curl-up, half, 145, 158
    dips, 55
    hamstring stretcher, 132-135, 148, 158
    jumping jacks, 122
    kicker, 152
    knee-to-nose kick, 153
    legovers, 127, 148
    low-back stretcher, 130, 148
    lower leg flexor, 141
    pull-ups, 53-54, 146-147
    push-ups, 143, 148
    quadricep strengthener, 139
    side leg raises, 128, 148
    side stretcher, 126, 148
    sitting tucks, 129
    sit-ups, 52-53, 144, 148, 158
    soleus stretcher, 137
    squat thrusts, 64, 141
    stride stretcher, 131, 148, 158
    toe touch, 124, 148
    trunk bender, 123
    trunk rotator, 125, 148
    weight training, 194-202
    see also Exercise

Fat cells, 237
Fatigue, 9, 25, 41, 103, 108, 210, 211
    posture and, 155-156
    see also Recovery
Fat measurements, 77-82, 238-240. See also
        Body fat; Weight control
Fats, 224-225
    in foods, 228-229

polyunsaturated, 224-225, 229
saturated, 225, 261-262
triglycerides, 35, 261-262
unsaturated, 225
Fatty acids, 224
Female, *see* Women
Fencing, 291
Fitness, components, 10-14, 119
    definition and components, 10-14
    designing personal program, 101-104
    evaluation of, 47-90
    lifetime sports and, 278-312
    prescription for, 93-101
    reasons for, 7-9, 14-17
    total, 93
    *see also* Evaluation; Physical fitness; *and*
        Workouts
Fixx, James, 266
Flexibility, defined, 12-13
    evaluation of, 57-60
    norms, for, 59-60
    sports and, 311
    trunk extension, 60
    trunk flexion, 59
    warm-up, 102
Food, caloric values of foods, 231-235
    seven food groups, 228-229
    *see also* Diet; Weight control
Fox, Sam, 271
Friedman, Meyer, 265

Girls, physical education curriculum, 6. *See also*
        Women
Girth measurements, 83-84. *See also* Body build;
        Body fat
Glucose, 223
Golf, 292
    caloric cost of, 245, 246
    cardiorespiratory fitness and, 99, 104, 293
Grip strength, 56
Gymnastics, 294

Half squats, 201
Hamstring stretcher, 132-135, 148, 158
Handball, 295
Health, cardiorespiratory fitness and, 13-14, 86
    exercise and, 6
    muscular, 14-15
    optimal, 10, 14
    spas, 117-118
Heart, arteriosclerosis, 258
    atherosclerosis, 258

cardiac output, 24-26, 28
cardiorespiratory endurance, 13-14
coronary arteries, 24, 258
myocardial infarction, 258
obesity and, 263
physiology of, 22-24
recovery test, 69-73
stroke volume, 25, 26
    *see also* Heart disease; Heart rate
Heart disease, activity and, 256-274
    cholesterol, 259, 260-262
    diabetes and, 263
    exercise, preventive measure, 163, 257, 266,
        269-272
    heredity and, 260
    hyperlipidemia, 262
    hypertension and, 260
    Irish brothers study, 270
    Korean war study, 258-259
    lipoproteins, 262
    population studies, 269-270
    Risko, 267-268
    risks, 9, 259-268
    Type A behavior, 265-266
Heart rate, formula for determining training rate, 94
    maximal, 28, 94, 164
    measurement of, 97-98
    recovery index, 71-72
    response during exercise, 26-27, 73-77,
        100-101
    response during recovery, 27
    resting, 22, 34, 94-97
    75% HR max, 94-98, 100, 103, 164, 175, 178,
        181, 183, 244, 310
    stationary bike test, 73-77
    step test, 69-73
    target, 103
    tests, 69-73, 73-77
    training heart rate, 92-99, 100, 103
Heat stroke, 249
Heel lifts, 200
Hemoglobin, defined, 22
    in women, 40
Heredity, heart disease and, 260
    maximal oxygen uptake and, 28-31
High blood pressure, *see* Hypertension
Hypertension, definition, 226, 260
    risk factor, 259-268
Hypertrophy, 11, 191

Ice skating, 296
Inactivity, 237, 240-241, 246

fatness and, 240
  heart disease risk and, 8-9, 266-267
Individual differences, AAHPER philosophy on, 6
  in regard to designing program, 101
  in regard to testing, 47-48
Injuries, avoiding, 107-109, 170, 177, 193
Interpretation of, profile sheets, 49, 50
  test results, 49-51
  T-scores, 50-51
Interval training, 207-210, 211-213
Isokinetics, 190, 202
Isometric strength, 190-191
Isotonic strength, 190-191

Jog-walk-jog program, 163-170
  regulating intensity, 100, 103, 164
Jogging, 104-105
  defined, 164
  estimating energy cost for, 243, 244, 245
  shoes, 106
  see also Running; Workouts
Judo, 298
Jumping jacks, 122

Karate, 299
Karvonen heart rate formula, 94
Kayaking, 286
Kostrubala, 37-38, 266
Krebs cycle, 33

Lactic acid, 25, 33, 98, 207
Lawrence, Ronald, 37
Legovers, 127, 148
Life-style, fullness of, 16-17, 271-272
  inactive, 9
  modern, 7-9
  optimal, 10
Low back pain, 155-158
  causes, 155
  exercises for, 158
  prevention, 155-158
Lungs, 24

Maximal oxygen uptake, 28-31, 34
  declines with age, 31
  relationship with "best effort" runs, 32, 66-68
  values, 29-31
  see also Aerobic capacity
Mayer, Jean, 224, 228, 246
Measurement, see Evaluation
Medical exam, 48, 93
Men, body fat, 77-82, 119-120

body girths, 83-84
  middle-aged training study, 39
  physique, 83
  weight training, 120
Menstruation, 40-41
Metabolic rate, BMR, 230
  calculations of, 230, 235-236
METS, 242, 244. See also Caloric cost
Michigan Heart Association, Risko game, 267-268
Minerals, 225-226
  in food, 228-229
Motor skill performance, defined, 13
  evaluation of, 61-66
Muscle, bulk in women, 11, 36, 39, 191-192
  fast twitch, 212
  fiber types, 212
  overload, 191
  slow twitch, 212
  soreness, 107-109
Muscle contraction, biochemical studies, 212
  physiology of, 32-33
Muscular endurance, defined, 11-12, 189
  sports and, 311
  see also Evaluation; Strength

Nutrients, carbohydrates, 223-224
  diet, 9-10, 228-229
  fats, 224-225
  food, 228-229
  high fat diet, 260-262
  minerals, 225-226
  protein, 222-223
  vitamins, 226
  water, 226
  see also Diet
Nutrition, caloric values of foods, 231-235
  definition of, 221
  salt in diet, 226
  Senate Committee on, 224, 227
  sugar in diet, 223-224
  see also Diet; Weight control

Obesity, 82, 237-240, 241
  as health hazard, 263-264
  walking program for, 177-178
  see also Weight control
Orienteering, 300
Overload, circuit training, 214
  interval training and, 207
  weight training, 190-192, 194-195
Overweight, 78, 177, 237. See also Body fat
Oxygen, aerobic capacity, 28-31

caloric equivalency and, 242
exercise requirements, 25
metabolic rate and, 230
role in muscle contraction, 32-33
Oxygen uptake, declines with age, 31
field tests for estimation of, 32, 66-68
maximal, 28-31
measurement of, 241
METS, 242-244
resting, 230, 235
*see also* Aerobic capacity

Palmer, Arnold, 292
Physical activity, heart disease and, 269-272
selection, 104-105
when and where to workout, 105-106
*see also* Exercises; Sports
Physical education, curriculum, 6
Physical fitness, benefits, 33-38
components, 10-14, 49, 119
defined, 10-14
fundamental reasons for, 14-17
prescription for, 92-112
profile summary sheets, 87, 88
rating of sports, 277, 310-312
total, 93
why?, 7-9
*see also* Exercise; Fitness; *and* Sports
Physical inactivity, *see* Inactivity
Physiology, basic, blood, 22
cardiorespiratory system, 22-25
fundamental knowledge of, 21
heart, 22-24
lungs, 24
Posture, 156-158
lifting, 157-158
sitting, 156
sleeping, 156
standing, 156
Power, definition, 189
Pregnancy, 41
Presidential Sports Award Program, 312-313
President's Council on Physical Fitness, award
program, 312-313
National Sports Survey, 118
Press, 196
bench, 197
Programs, *see* Training methods; Workouts
Protein, 222-223
in foods, 228-229
Psychological benefits from exercise, 36-38
Pull-up, 53-54, 146-147

Punishment, approach to exercise, 6
Push-ups, 143, 148

Racquetball, 302
Recovery, after workout, 103-104
cool down, 103-104
during workout, 98
heart rate, 25-28
interval training and, 208-209
step-test, 69-73
Respiratory system, structure of, 24
Ribisl, Paul, 68
Risk factors, heart disease, 9, 259-268
Risko, 267-268
Rope skipping, 142
Rosenman, Ray H., 265
Rowing, 184
bent-over, 200
upright, 199
Running, continuous, 210-213, 244-245
distance, 290
interval, 207-210
shoes, 106
tests, 32
*see also* Jogging

Saltin, Bengt, 212
Scuba diving, 303
Senate Committee, 224, 227
Sex differences, of men and women to exercise,
28, 39-40
oxygen uptake, 29-30
strength and muscular endurance, 39, 191-192
training responses, 39-40
Sheehan, George, 37
Shoes, jogging, 106
Side leg raises, 128, 148
Side stretcher, 126, 148
Sitting tucks, 129
Sit-ups, 52-53, 144, 148, 158
Skating, ice, 296
Skiing, Alpine, 278
cross-country, 184-185, 288
water, 309
Skill, measurement of, 60-64
motor performance defined, 13
Skin diving, 304
Skinfold measurements with calipers, 78-79,
238-240
norms, 82, 239-240
*see also* Body fat
Skipping rope, 142

Sleep, 37
  need for, 9
  posture, 156
Sloan, A. W., 78
Smoking, emphysema, 264
  heart disease, 264
Sports, 276-312
  contributions to physical fitness, 277-278
  lifetime activities, 277-278
  motivator to exercise, 277
  Presidents award program, 312-313
  rating charts, 310-312
  rating fitness potential, 310-312
  selection, 104-105, 310
  tables, 311-312
  team, 278
  *see also each sport as listed*
Squat thrusts, 64, 141
Step-test, norms, 72-73
  procedure, 70-71
  *see also* Heart rate; Recovery
Strength, defined, 11, 189
  grip, 56
  improvement of, 189-190, 194-195
  isokinetics, 190, 202
  isometric, 190-191
  isotonic, 190-191
  sports and, 311
  women and, 11, 39, 191, 192
  *see also* Muscle; Weight training
Stride stretcher, 131, 148
Stroke volume, 25, 34, 76
Sugar, 223
  blood, 223
  refined, 223-224
Surfing, 305
Sweating, 93, 102, 119
  steam room, 248
  wearing rubber suit, 106, 248
Swimming, 99, 104, 105, 306
  compared with jogging, 177
  training, 174-177, 210

Tennis, 61, 99-100, 104, 307
Tension, 7, 265-266, 271-272
Test, agility, 62
  body build, 83-84
  body fat, 77-82
  cardiorespiratory endurance, 32, 65-77
  flexibility, 58-60
  heart rate, 69-77
  medical exam, 48, 93

muscular endurance, 51-56
  power, 63
  step test, 70-73
  strength, 51-57
  treadmill stress test, 28-29
  *see also* Evaluation
Testing, classification charts, of results, 49-51
  interpretation and, 49-51
  motivation, 47-48
  purpose of, 47-49
  self-testing, 47-49
  shortcomings of, 47
  test battery, explanation, 49
Toe touch, 124, 148
Training effect, 7, 25-27, 34, 163, 170
Training methods, bicycle, 170-174
  circuit training, 213-216
  continuous, 210-213
  interval, 207-210, 211-213
  jog-walk-jog, 163-170
  prescription factors, 93-104
  stationary bike, 178-181
  swimming, 173-177
  walking, 177-178
  weight training, 188-204
  *see also* Exercise
Triglycerides, 261
Trunk bends, 123, 148
Trunk extension, 60
Trunk flexion, 59
Trunk rotator, 125, 148
T-score, conversion tables, men, 327-329
    women, 324-326
  *see also* Classification tables
Type-A behavior, 265-266

Ullyot, Joan, 39
Upright rowing, 199

Vertical jump, 63
Vitamins, 226
  in foods, 228-229

Walking, 177-178
Warm-up, avoiding injury, 102
  defined, 102
  importance of, 102, 163
  routine for, 148
  weight training, 195
  *see also* Exercises
Water, loss and dehydration, 248-249
  as nutrient, 226

Water ballet, 307
Water skiing, 309
Weight control, 36, 221
    approximating your desired weight, 250-251
    caloric cost and, 242-246
    estimating desired weight, 250-251
    lifetime concept of, 251
    misconceptions of, 246-249
    plan for, 249-251
    role of exercise in, 240-246
    spot reducing, 117, 247
    see also Body fat; Obesity
Weight reduction, by exercise, 240, 249-251
    plan for, 249-251
    by spot reducing, 247
    by sweating, 248-249
Weight tables, inadequacy of, 238-240
Weight training, 188-204
    basic equipment, 192
    beginning program, 194-195
    cardiorespiratory fitness and, 100, 192, 195
    exercises, 195-202
    principles-procedures, 193-194
    program, 192-195
    safety precautions, 193
    strength development, 11, 190-194
    terminology, 192
    women and, 11, 36, 39, 191-192
Wilmore, Jack, 191, 192
Women, energy needs for, 235
    biomechanics of running, 109
    bra selection, 106-107
    exercises for, 149-154

girths, recommended, 83-84
gynecological considerations, 40-41
heart disease, 257, 259
hemoglobin and, 40
increasing breast size, 119
injuries, 107-109
jogging, energy cost for, 244
losing weight, 119
maximal oxygen uptake values for, 30-31
measuring fat and girths, 77-85, 119
menstruation, 40
middle-aged training study, 39
muscle mass development, 11, 36, 39, 191-192
pregnancy, childbirth, 41
response to physical training, 6, 39
strength development and, 11, 36
weight training, 191-192
Workouts, bicycle, 173-174
    circuit, 215
    continuous training, 210-211
    exercises, basic conditioning, 117-154
    interval training, 208-209
    jog-walk-jog, 166-169
    modifying your workout, 100, 103, 164-165
    stationary bike, 180
    swimming, 176
    walking, 177-178
    warm-up, 148
    weight training, 194-195
    see also Exercise; Training methods

Yoga, 247